D0222083

THOMSON DELMAR LEARNING'S
CASE STUDY SERIES

Pediatrics

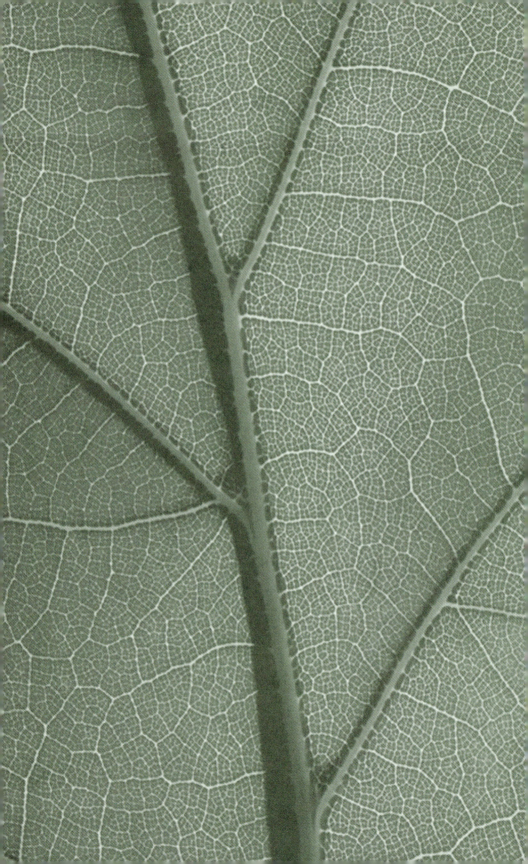

THOMSON DELMAR LEARNING'S CASE STUDY SERIES

Pediatrics

Bonita E. Broyles
RN, BSN, MA, PhD

Instructor
ADN PROGRAM, PIEDMONT
COMMUNITY COLLEGE,
NORTH CAROLINA

THOMSON
———✦———
DELMAR LEARNING

Australia   Canada   Mexico   Singapore   Spain   United Kingdom   United States

2/07

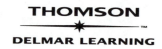

THOMSON
TM
DELMAR LEARNING

Thomson Delmar Learning's Case Study Series: Pediatrics
by Bonita Broyles

**Vice President,
Health Care Business Unit:**
William Brottmiller

Editorial Director:
Cathy L. Esperti

Executive Editor:
Matthew Kane

Developmental Editor:
Maria D'Angelico

Editorial Assistant:
Michelle Leavitt

Marketing Director:
Jennifer McAvey

Channel Manager:
Tamara Caruso

Marketing Coordinator:
Michele Gleason

Production Director:
Carolyn Miller

Production Editor:
Jack Pendleton

COPYRIGHT © 2006 by Thomson Delmar Learning, a part of The Thomson Corporation. Thomson, the Star logo, and Delmar Learning are trademarks used herein under license.

Printed in United States of America
1 2 3 4 5 6 7 XXX 08 07 06 05

For more information, contact Thomson Delmar Learning, 5 Maxwell Drive, Clifton Park, NY 12065-2919
Or you can visit our Internet site at http://www.delmarlearning.com

ALL RIGHTS RESERVED. No part of this work covered by the copyright hereon may be reproduced or used in any form or by any means— graphic, electronic, or mechanical, including photocopying, recording, taping, Web distribution or informa- tion storage and retrieval systems— without the written permission of the publisher.

For permission to use material from this text or product, contact us by
Tel (800) 730-2214
Fax (800) 730-2215
www.thomsonrights.com

Library of Congress Cataloging-in-Publication Data

Broyles, Bonita E.
    Pediatrics/Bonita E. Broyles.
        p. ; cm. —
    (Thomson Delmar learning's case study series)
    Includes bibliographical references and index.
    ISBN 1-4018-2633-4
    1. Pediatric nursing—Case studies.
    [DNLM: 1. Pediatric Nursing— Case Reports. WY 159 B885p 2006]
    I. Title. II. Series.
    RJ245.B793 2006
    618.92'00231—dc22

    2005011105

    ISBN 1-4018-2633-4

Notice to the Reader

Contents

Reviewers

Jane H. Barnsteiner RN, PhD, FAAN
Professor of Pediatric Nursing
University of Pennsylvania School of Nursing
Philadelphia, Pennsylvania

Diana Jacobson MS, RN, CPNO
Faculty Associate
Arizona State University, College of Nursing
Tempe, Arizona

Nancy Oldenburg RN, MS, CPNP
Clinical Instructor
Northern Illinois University
DeKalb, Illinois

Deborah J. Persell MSN, RN, CPNP
Assistant Professor
Arkansas State University
Jonesboro, Arkansas

JoAnne Solchany RN, ARNP, PhD, CS
Assistant Professor, Family & Child Nursing
University of Washington
Seattle, Washington

Preface

Thomson Delmar Learning's Case Studies Series was created to encourage nurses to bridge the gap between content knowledge and clinical application. The products within the series represent the most innovative and comprehensive approach to nursing case studies ever developed. Each title has been authored by experienced nurse educators and clinicians who understand the complexity of nursing practice as well as the challenges of teaching and learning. All of the cases are based on real-life clinical scenarios and demand thought and "action" from the nurse. Each case brings the user into the clinical setting, and invites him or her to utilize the nursing process while considering all of the variables that influence the client's condition and the care to be provided. Each case also represents a unique set of variables, to offer a breadth of learning experiences and to capture the reality of nursing practice. To gauge the progression of a user's knowledge and critical thinking ability, the cases have been categorized by difficulty level. Every section begins with basic cases and proceeds to more advanced scenarios, thereby presenting opportunities for learning and practice for both students and professionals. All of the cases have undergone expert review to ensure that as many variables as possible are represented in a truly realistic manner and that each case reflects consistency with realities of modern nursing practice.

How to Use This Book

Every case begins with a table of variables that are encountered in practice, and that must be understood by the nurse in order to provide appropriate care to the client. Categories of variables include age; gender; setting; ethnicity; pre-existing conditions; coexisting conditions; cultural, communication disability, socioeconomic, spiritual, pharmacological, psychosocial, legal, ethical, prioritization, and delegation considerations; and alternative therapy. If a case involves a variable that is considered to have a significant impact on care, the specific variable is included in the table. This allows the user an "at a glance" view of the issues that will need to be considered to provide care to the client in the scenario. The table of variables is followed by a presentation of the case, including the history of the client, current condition, clinical setting, and professionals involved. A series of questions follows each case that ask the user to consider how she would handle the issues presented within the scenario. Suggested answers and rationales are provided for remediation and discussion.

Organization

The cases are grouped into parts based on topics. Within each part, cases are organized by difficulty level from easy, to moderate, to difficult. This classification is somewhat subjective, but they are based upon a developed standard. In general, difficulty level has been determined by the number of variables that impact the case and the complexity of the client's condition. Colored tabs are used to allow the user to distinguish the difficulty levels more easily. A comprehensive table of variables is also provided for reference, to allow the user to quickly select cases containing a particular variable of care.

Praise for Thomson Delmar Learning's Case Study Series

I would recommend this book to my undergraduate students. This would be a required book for graduate students in nursing education, women's health, or maternal-child programs.

—Patricia Posey-Goodwin, M.S.N, R.N., Ed.D (c)
Assistant Professor,
University of West Florida

This text does an excellent job of reflecting the complexity of nursing practice.

—Vicki Nees, RNC, MSN, APRN-BC
Associate Professor,
Ivy Tech State College

. . . the case studies are very comprehensive and allow the under-graduate student an opportunity to apply knowledge gained in the classroom to a potentially real clinical situation.

—TAMELLA LIVENGOOD, APRN, BC, MSN, FNP
Nursing Faculty,
Northwestern Michigan College

I commend the effort to include the impact of illness on the growth and development of the child, on the family's cohesiveness and on the subsequent health problems that will affect the child in years to come. Inclusion of questions that focus on the nurse's perceptions, biases and beliefs are extremely important when training nurses to provide comprehensive care . . . Often one system illness will affect another health system and this has been demonstrated numerous times [in this text].

—DIANA JACOBSON, MS, RN, CPNP
Faculty Associate,
Arizona State University College of Nursing

These cases and how you have approached them definitely stimu-late the students to use critical-thinking skills. I thought the ques-tions asked really pushed the students to think deeply and thoroughly.

—JOANNE SOLCHANY, PhD, ARNP, RN, CS
Assistant Professor,
Family & Child Nursing,
University of Washington, Seattle.

The use of case studies is pedagogically sound and very appealing to students and instructors. I think that some instructors avoid them because of the challenge of case development. You have pro-vided the material for them.

—NANCY L. OLDENBURG, RN, MS, CPNP
Clinical Instructor,
Northern Illinois University

[The author] has done an excellent job of assisting students to engage in critical thinking. I am very impressed with the cases, questions and content. I rarely ask that students buy more than one pediatrics book . . . but, in this instance, I can't wait until this book is published.

—DEBORAH J. PERSELL, MSN, RN, CPNP
Assistant Professor,
Arkansas State University

This is a groundbreaking book that ... will be appropriate for undergraduate pediatric courses as well as a variety of graduate programs . . . One of the most impressive features is the variety of cases that cover situations from primary care through critical care and rehabilitation. The cases are presented to develop and assess critical-thinking skills . . . All cases are framed within a comprehensive presentation of physical findings, stimulating critical thinking about pathophysiology, developmental considerations, and family systems. This book should be a required text for all undergraduate and graduate nursing programs and should be well-received by faculty.

—JANE H. BARNSTEINER, PhD, RN, FAAN
Professor of Pediatric Nursing,
University of Pennsylvania School of Nursing

Note from the Author

These case studies were designed to assist nursing students of all levels develop and strengthen their critical thinking skills to provide the best care for this very special client population. I have thoroughly enjoyed writing this work of heart.

About the Author

Dr. Broyles began her nursing career in 1968, working as a student nursing assistant while pursuing her Bachelor of Science degree in nursing from The Ohio State University in Columbus, Ohio. She graduated with her BSN in 1970 and continued for the next 13 years staffing and teaching on obstetrics and gynecology. From 1972 to 1976, she taught in the Associate Degree Nursing Education program at Columbus Technical Institute (which is now Columbus State). During her 5-year position as Patient Teaching and Discharge Planning Coordinator for Obstetrics and Gynecology at Mt. Carmel Medical Center in Columbus (1976–1981), she published her first professional writing. At this juncture, she decided to expand both her mind and nursing skills into the medical-surgical arena of nursing where she has staffed and taught nursing since that time to present. With her husband, Roger, she moved to North Carolina in 1985. She has been an educator in the nursing education department of Piedmont Community College in Roxboro, North Carolina since 1986 and is currently the course coordinator for Maternal-Child Nursing (teaching the pediatric component of the course), Adult Nursing II, and Pharmacology. Dr. Broyles received her Master of Arts in Educational Media from North Carolina Central University in 1988, and her Doctorate of Education in Adult Education from LaSalle University in 1996. Her dissertation research concerned critical thinking in Associate Degree Nursing Students and was the largest study published on this topic. In 2004, Dr. Broyles received her PhD from St. Regis University with further study in adult education. Dr. Broyles has published nursing texts in the areas of pediatrics, medical-surgical nursing, and pharmacology.

Acknowledgments

The author wishes to express her appreciation to all who contributed to the development of these cases. Without the love, support, encouragement, and diligence of my husband Roger this project as with those past would not be the success I believe this will be. I also thank the many friends and colleagues who helped me through their love, support, encouragement, and expertise. Thank you, Mama Lou, Papa Joe, Pat, Alisa, Kelly, and Colman.

The author also wishes to acknowledge the Associate Degree Nursing Education students who serve as continuing inspiration to produce student-friendly textbooks that help them learn this most important content for their safe nursing practice.

For the opportunity to be involved in this project, the author wishes to thank the people at Thomson Delmar Learning for their support, encouragement, and editorial guidance during the writing of the Pediatric Case Studies. Special thanks go to Matt Kane, who continues to believe in me as a nursing author, and to Michelle Leavitt, whose enthusiasm and flexibility helped make this project so enjoyable.

Finally, the author wishes to thank the reviewers of this work for their time and expertise evident in their constructive comments and suggestions. Having been a book reviewer for 5 years, the author appreciates the time and effort of the reviewers as they share their knowledge and expertise to help make this edition a worthy educational tool.

Bonita E. Broyles

Comprehensive Table of Variables

Case Study	Gender	Age	Setting	Ethnicity	Cultural Considerations	Preexisting Conditions	Coexisting Conditions	Communication	Disability	Socioeconomic	Spiritual	Pharmacologic	Psychosocial	Legal	Ethical	Alternative Therapy	Prioritization	Delegation
Part One: The Digestive and Urinary Systems																		
1	M	11 months	Community clinic	Black American		×				×		×	×					×
2	M	18 months	Home/hospital	Asian American	Asian			×		×		×	×			×	×	×
3	M	5	Hospital	Spanish American	Hispanic	×						×	×					
4	M	13 months	Hospital	White American		×						×	×		×		×	×
Part Two: The Respiratory System																		
1	M	4	Emergency room	Asian American								×	×				×	×
2	M	7	School	Native American		×	×					×	×					×
3	F	6 weeks	Hospital	White American		×						×	×					
Part Three: The Cardiovascular System and the Blood																		
1	F	13	Home/health care provider's office	White American		×							×					
2	F	7	Clinic	Mediterranean				×				×	×					×
3	M	8	Hospital	White American						×			×	×	×			
Part Four: The Skeletal, Muscular, and Integumentary Systems																		
1	F	8 months	Hospital	Black American									×					
2	M	5 and 8	Hospital/emergency department/home/clinic	White American								×	×				×	×
3	F	9	Hospital	Black American		×	×	×	×			×	×					×

Part Five: The Nervous and Endocrine Systems

1	F	2½	Clinic	Spanish American
2	M	4 months	Hospital	Black American
3	M	neonate	Hospital	White American

Part Six: The Lymphatic System

1	F	4 months	Clinic	White American
2	M	4 weeks	Community/hospital	East African
3	M	10	Home	White American

Part Seven: The Reproductive System

1	F	15	Clinic	White American

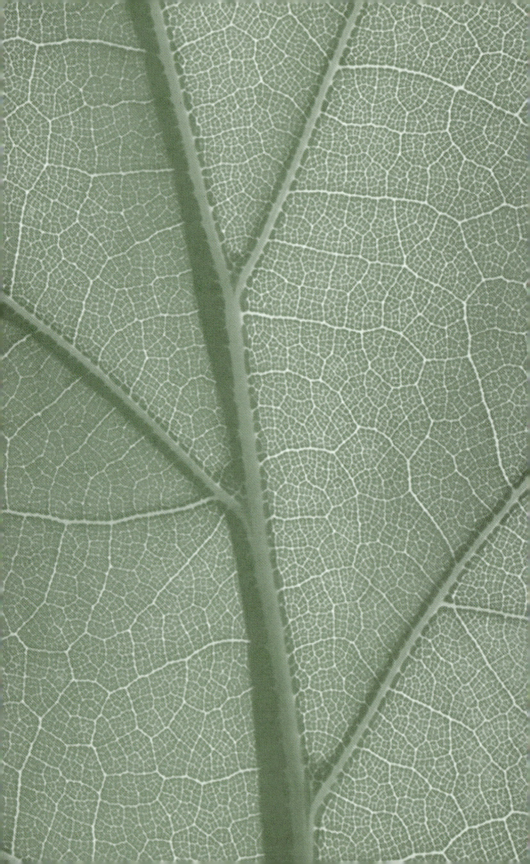

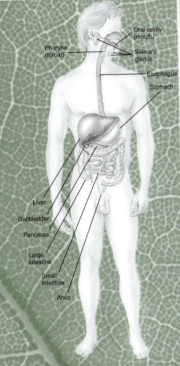

PART ONE

Oral cavity (mouth)

Pharynx (throat)

Salivary glands

Esophagus

Stomach

Liver

Gallbladder

Pancreas

Large intestine

Small intestine

Anus

Digestive system Mouth, pharynx, esophagus, stomach, small intestine, large intestine, salivary glands, pancreas, gallbladder, and liver.

The Digestive and Urinary Systems

CASE STUDY 1

Timothy

GENDER

M

AGE

11 months old

SETTING

- Community clinic

ETHNICITY

- Black American

CULTURAL CONSIDERATIONS

PREEXISTING CONDITIONS

- No well-baby appointments

COEXISTING CONDITIONS

COMMUNICATION

DISABILITY

SOCIOECONOMIC

- Lower socioeconomic

SPIRITUAL

PHARMACOLOGIC

PSYCHOSOCIAL

- Single teenage mother

LEGAL

ETHICAL

ALTERNATIVE THERAPY

PRIORITIZATION

DELEGATION

- Client teaching

THE DIGESTIVE SYSTEM

Level of difficulty: Easy

Overview: This case requires knowledge of growth and development, nutrition, failure-to-thrive (FTT), as well as an understanding of the client's background, personal situation, and mother–child attachment relationship.

Client Profile

Timothy is an 11-month-old infant who lives with his 16-year-old mother and his grandmother in an urban apartment. His mother, Fascia, has stayed at home with Timothy since his birth, but plans to return to school this coming fall. His grandmother works 12-hour shifts to support her daughter and grandson. Because of her mother's work schedule, Fascia has little guidance at home. Fascia and her mother bring Timothy in to the clinic for his first visit because he needs a physical and "shots" so he can be enrolled in daycare when Fascia returns to school in a month.

Case Study

While taking his history, the nurse finds that Timothy has generalized weakness and is cachexiac. He weighs in the 5th percentile for his height and age. The nurse notes that Timothy has not received his 2-, 4-, or 6-month immunizations. Fascia tells the nurse that she didn't know he needed "shots" until she and her mother tried to enroll him in daycare. She further tells the nurse that when Timothy cries, she feeds him but he usually drinks only "half a bottle (8 oz)" of cow's milk at each feeding. She feeds him table food when he is up at a time she is eating. Fascia tells the nurse that Timothy is a "good baby" who doesn't cry much and sleeps most of the time. He sits up by himself but hasn't started crawling. Fascia keeps him in his playpen when he is awake and he reaches and grasps objects with the palms of his hands on his cradle gym. He says "mama" and "bye-bye." Fascia says she doesn't hold Timothy "much because I don't want to spoil him."

Questions

1. Discuss the significance of Timothy's clinical manifestations.

2. What other assessment data would be helpful for the nurse to have to prepare Timothy's care plan?

3. What are Timothy's risk factors for failure to thrive (FTT)?

4. Compare organic, nonorganic, and idiopathic FTT.

5. Discuss the usual diagnostic tests used to determine which type of FTT a child has.

6. What are the priorities of care for Timothy?

7. Discuss the impact of a diagnosis of nonorganic failure to thrive on Timothy's growth and development.

8. Discuss the potential long-term effects of FTT.

9. Would a multidisciplinary team approach be beneficial to Timothy and his family? Who should be involved in this team?

10. Discuss the teaching priorities for Fascia prior to taking Timothy home from the clinic.

Questions and Suggested Answers

1. **Discuss the significance of Timothy's clinical manifestations.** Timothy's weight places him within the definition of failure to thrive. He is developmentally delayed, as evidenced by his mother's report of his activities. Most infants can crawl and pull themselves up by the age of 8–9 months. His sitting is consistent with the developmental stage of a 6- to 7-month-old. His fine motor skills of reaching and grasping objects with the palms of the hands represent the fine motor skills of a 4- to 5-month-old. His vocabulary is consistent with that of a 7-month-old.

2. **What other assessment data would be helpful for the nurse to have to prepare Timothy's care plan?**
   a. Birth weight and height
   b. Gestational age at birth
   c. Daily intake and output
   d. Condition of his anterior fontanel
   e. Skin assessment
   f. Heart sounds
   g. Lung sounds
   h. Bowel sounds
   i. Daily interactions between mother and child
   j. Developmental markers

3. **What are Timothy's risk factors for failure to thrive (FTT)?**
   a. Adolescent mother
   b. Lack of knowledge about infant nutrition
   c. Lack of knowledge about well-baby care including immunizations
   d. Inaccurate knowledge about "spoiling" an infant
   e. Little supervision by grandmother because of work schedule
   f. Possible money issues for proper nutrition

4. **Compare organic, nonorganic, and idiopathic FTT.** Organic failure to thrive is caused by physiologic factors that interfere with an infant's ability to ingest and/or utilize nutrition. These factors include congenital heart defects that result in fatigue; cystic fibrosis; celiac disease resulting in malabsorption; neurological disorders including microcephaly; renal failure; gastroesophageal reflux (GER); and acquired immunodeficiency syndrome. Oral–motor difficulties in the baby also can lead to organic failure to thrive. Nonorganic FTT is caused by psychosocial factors including lack of parental/caregiver knowledge of nutritional needs of children; lack of bonding related to mother's developmental level or separation from the infant during critical early infancy period; child neglect or abuse. Idiopathic FTT occurs with no definable cause. All types of FTT result in weight below the 3rd to 5th percentile for age and height.

5. Discuss the usual diagnostic tests used to determine which type of FTT a child has. The initial diagnostic tests are focused on determining or ruling out the presence of physical causes. These include physical examination to identify or rule out congenital defects including heart defects; sweat chloride for cystic fibrosis; developmental screening to determine achievement of milestones; bone scan to determine bone length, thickness, and epiphyseal development; chest x-ray for pulmonary dysfunction; urinalysis and blood chemistries for renal and urinary function; complete blood count for anemia and/or chronic or systemic infections; fecal examination for saccharide deficiencies, milk intolerance, internal bleeding, parasitic infections, and malabsorption; thyroid screening; electrocardiography for cardiac anomalies; gastrointestinal series for obstruction; bowel and muscle biopsies to rule out Hirschsprung disease, celiac disease, and muscular dystrophy; and serum testing for lead toxicity.

6. What is the goal of treatment for Timothy? What are his nursing priorities of care? The goal of treatment is to provide sufficient calories, macronutrients, and micronutrients for Timothy to experience rapid growth to the level appropriate for his age. Providing his mother and grandmother education about immunizations and his developmental needs also is needed. The nursing priorities of care include:
   a. Imbalanced nutrition: less than body requirements related to inadequate nutritional intact
   b. Risk for injury, complications related to inadequate nutrition
   c. Delayed growth and development related to parental deficient knowledge and imbalanced nutrition
   d. Deficient knowledge related to Timothy's nutritional needs, normal growth, and development

7. Discuss the impact of a diagnosis of nonorganic failure to thrive on Timothy's growth and development. Nonorganic FTT is the result of psychosocial factors. The fact that Fascia is giving Timothy cow's milk indicates a knowledge deficit regarding what is appropriate for infant feedings. Infants should receive formula designed for infant consumption until they are 12 months of age. Giving cow's milk to an infant can result in gastrointestinal bleeding and anemia because the infant's GI system cannot digest the proteins in cow's milk. Fascia's comment about not holding Timothy much because she didn't want to spoil him also indicates a lack of knowledge about infant needs. Infants cannot be spoiled because this behavior requires deliberate actions resulting from cognitive functioning beyond the level of an infant. Infants cry because they have a need—hunger, discomfort, need for tactile stimulation, overstimulation. The scenario implies that Timothy does not receive much stimulation which is necessary for cognitive and sensory development. His delayed verbal development may be the result of inadequate verbal stimulation. Developmental delays may be temporary if the cause is treated or permanent if it is not.

8. **Discuss the potential long-term effects of FTT.** Failure to thrive can have long-term effects that impact the immune system, the gastrointestinal system, nervous system, and his growth and development.
   a. Immune system
      (1) repeated respiratory infections and otitis media
   b. Gastrointestinal system
      (1) iron-deficiency anemia
      (2) lead absorption secondary to deficient iron and calcium intake
      (3) constipation and bowel obstruction
      (4) repeated gastrointestinal infections
   c. Developmental delays
   d. Insufficient organ development in all systems

9. **Would a multidisciplinary team approach be beneficial to Timothy and his family? Who should be involved in this team?** A multidisciplinary team approach would be very helpful in this situation. A social worker could assist with finding available programs to purchase appropriate nutrition for Timothy (WIC), financial assistance through Medicaid, child-care funding so Fascia can return to school. A child-life specialist could provide information and assistance in Fascia receiving classes about child care, infant nutrition, infant growth and development needs. A nutritionist could help plan high-calorie, high-carbohydrate, high–fat, and protein intake to facilitate Timothy "catching up" to his desired weight and development for height and age. The health care provider and the nurse also are important components of the team. A home health referral would be a way to monitor Timothy's nutritional progress and Fascia's learning progress.

10. **Discuss the teaching priorities for Fascia prior to taking Timothy home from the clinic.**
    a. Information concerning normal growth and development of infants
    b. Dietary needs specified by the nutritionist
    c. A written schedule for feedings including specific foods and amounts
    d. Need to interface with infant throughout the day
    e. Importance of Fascia having time away from Timothy so she can develop as an adolescent
    f. Stress that feedings should be a relaxing time
    g. Need to monitor intake and output
    h. Information concerning referrals and names and phone numbers of contacts
    i. Importance of regular follow-up in clinic

j. Immunization schedule (this will begin as a make-up schedule until Timothy is current with his immunizations)
k. Encourage Fascia and her mother to ask questions, providing them with phone numbers of contact individuals
l. Provide sufficient time for Fascia and her mother to ask questions, ensuring they receive answers
m. Document teaching and Fascia and her mother's response

References

Centers for Disease Control. *http://www.cdc.gov*

Daniels, R. (2002). *Delmar's manual of laboratory and diagnostic tests.* Clifton Park, NY: Thomson Delmar Learning.

eMedicine—Failure to Thrive: Article by Reda W. Bassali, MBChB. *http://www.emedicine.com*

Failure to Thrive. *http://www.kidshealth.org*

Medline Plus: Failure to Thrive. *http://www.nlm.nih.gov*

North American Nursing Diagnosis Association (2005). *Nursing diagnoses: Definitions & classifications, 2005–2006.* Philadelphia: NANDA.

Potts, N. and Mandleco, B. (2002). *Pediatric nursing: Caring for children and their families.* Clifton Park, NY: Thomson Delmar Learning, pp. 1196–1198.

Wong, D.L., Perry, S.E., and Hockenberry, M.J. (2002). *Maternal child nursing care* (2nd ed.). St. Louis: Mosby, pp. 869–873.

Colman

GENDER

M

AGE

18 months old

SETTING

- Home/hospital

ETHNICITY

- Asian American

CULTURAL CONSIDERATIONS

- Asian

PREEXISTING CONDITIONS

COEXISTING CONDITIONS

COMMUNICATION

DISABILITY

SOCIOECONOMIC

SPIRITUAL

PHARMACOLOGIC

- Acetaminophen (Tylenol)
- *N*-acetylcysteine (Mucomyst)

PSYCHOSOCIAL

- Parental anxiety

LEGAL

ETHICAL

ALTERNATIVE THERAPY

- Herbal remedies

PRIORITIZATION

- Emergency situation

DELEGATION

MODERATE

THE DIGESTIVE SYSTEM

Level of difficulty: Moderate

Overview: This case requires knowledge of poisoning, growth and development, traditional and alternative medications, as well as an understanding of the client's background, personal situation, and parent–child relationship.

Client Profile

Colman is an 18-month-old toddler who lives with his parents and 4-year-old brother in a northeastern city. Colman's mother, Mrs. Chan, stays at home with the children while their father operates a local restaurant. Colman has been walking since he was 10 months old and he and his brother spend most of the day playing with age-appropriate toys. Colman is very active and loves to pretend he is cooking like his mother. He has a set of play dishes and a small table and chairs where he and his brother pretend they are making dinner. Colman loves to open cabinets and climb in them. His parents have purchased child-proof locks for the cabinets, but haven't installed them yet.

Case Study

While Colman's brother is attending a neighborhood birthday party at a friend's house, Colman is playing with his playdough, making "dinner." He goes into the bathroom and finds the chewable acetaminophen his mother keeps in the medicine cabinet to be used when her children experience fevers. The acetaminophen 80-mg tablets are in a 250-count plastic bottle. He takes the medicine to his table and begins to eat his "play candy." His mother returns from the kitchen to find Colman vomiting, pale, and lethargic. She picks up Colman and runs carrying him three blocks to the emergency department of the medical center. She appears very anxious and screaming "My baby's been poisoned!"

Questions

1. What priority assessment should the nurse make as Colman and his mother enter the emergency department?

2. Discuss the significance of Colman's level of growth and development and his risk for poisoning.

3. What are the complications related to the ingestion of poisons in children?

4. What are the priorities of care for Colman on admission?

5. Discuss the nursing goals for Colman related to his priorities of care.

6. Colman's oxygen saturation is 89%. What actions should the nurse take?

7. A nasogastric tube is placed and Colman is prescribed *N*-acetylcysteine (Mucomyst) per nasogastric tube. Discuss the purpose of this treatment.

8. Colman is transferred to the pediatric intensive care unit (PICU) of the hospital and placed on mechanical ventilation. Discuss the rationale for this treatment.

9. The health care provider prescribes serum liver enzymes be drawn and schedules Colman for a liver biopsy. Discuss the rationale for these prescriptions and the nursing responsibilities following Colman's liver biopsy.

10. You overhear Mrs. Chan's phone conversation to consider using Chinese herbal remedies to speed Colman's recovery. Discuss the importance of the nurse's intervention regarding this situation.

11. Colman recovers and is to be discharged this morning. Discuss the teaching priorities for Colman's parents.

Questions and Suggested Answers

1. What priority assessment should the nurse make as Colman and his mother enter the emergency department? The nurse's first priority assessment is to determine the state of Colman's airway, breathing, and circulation (ABCs). The assessment must be accurate and rapid with the initial focus on his respiratory function and his cardiovascular integrity. During the assessment, the nurse must take a history to determine what substance Colman ingested as that is one of the indicators for how he needs to be treated. The nurse focuses on Colman's neurological status and then completes her rapid head-to-toe assessment and collaborates with the health care provider with her findings.

2. Discuss the significance of Colman's level of growth and development and his risk for poisoning. Colman is a toddler and toddlers are pursuing the task of autonomy versus shame and doubt. They are becoming more mobile and beginning to develop independence from parents although they don't usually stray very far. Toddlers spend most of their time playing and investigating their environment with their new gross motor skills. Because their sense of their abilities is far greater than their actual competencies, toddlers are constantly at risk for injury. Their need to investigate leaves them in danger of poisonings, water injuries, and pedestrian accidents. They must be closely monitored, but need to be allowed to pursue their autonomy.

3. What are the complications related to the ingestion of poisons in children? The complications are related to the substance ingested but include upper gastrointestinal tissue destruction (corrosives), central nervous system depression, liver failure (*acetaminophen*), metabolic acidosis or alkalosis, shock, and death, usually from respiratory failure.

4. What are the priorities of care for Colman on admission? (Including but not limited to)
   a. Risk for deficient fluid volume related to effects of ingested substances, treatment modalities, and decreased oral intake
   b. Risk for injury, liver failure related to ingestion of acetaminophen
   c. Anxiety (parental) related to sudden hospitalization and emergency aspect of condition
   d. Deficient knowledge related to growth and development and risk for poisoning, treatment, and home care

5. Discuss the nursing goals for Colman related to his priorities of care.
   a. Colman will maintain fluid and electrolyte volume as evidenced by serum electrolyte levels within normal limits and balanced fluid volume.
   b. Colman will not experience liver failure as evidenced by liver enzymes and liver biopsy within normal limits.

c. Colman's parents will verbalize their feelings and concerns and demonstrate characteristics of decreased anxiety.

d. Colman's parents will demonstrate an understanding of Colman's condition, treatment, growth and development, and poison safety

6. Colman's oxygen saturation is 89%. What actions should the nurse take? The first action of the nurse is to assess Colman's color and respiratory and neurological status as a means of confirming the accuracy of the pulse oximetry. The pulse oximetry sensor should be checked to be sure it is properly applied. The nurse needs to inform the health care provider of her findings and prepare to administer oxygen to Colman. Oxygen prescriptions now are usually written to administer oxygen to maintain oxygen saturations >94%. The normal range for oxygen saturation is 95% to 100%.

7. A nasogastric tube is placed and Colman is prescribed *N*-acetylcysteine (Mucomyst) per nasogastric tube. Discuss the purpose of this treatment. The standard of care for acetaminophen poisoning is activated charcoal because "oral activated charcoal avidly adsorbs acetaminophen and should be administered if the patient presents within 1–2 hours of ingestion or later" (Farrell, 2004). *N*-acetylcysteine is the antidote for acetaminophen poisoning and acts by preventing the formation and accumulation of a toxic metabolite, *N*-acetyl-*p*-benzoquinone-imine (NAPQI), the substance primarily indicated as the cause of acetaminophen-induced hepatotoxicity, the primary complication associated with acetaminophen poisoning. *N*-acetylcysteine usually is administered per nasogastric tube because of its characteristic offensive sulfur odor.

8. Colman is transferred to the pediatric intensive care unit (PICU) of the hospital and placed on mechanical ventilation. Discuss the rationale for this treatment. Ingestion of excessive amounts of *acetaminophen* can cause depression of the central nervous center including the respiratory center. This effect will cause an ineffective breathing pattern with resultant impaired gas exchange. Mechanical ventilation provides for adequate gas exchange until the effects of the drug are decreased to the point that Colman's normal respiratory effort and ability to exchange oxygen and carbon dioxide returns.

9. The health care provider prescribes serum liver enzymes be drawn and schedules Colman for a liver biopsy. Discuss the rationale for these prescriptions and the nursing responsibilities following Colman's liver biopsy. The major complication associated with acetaminophen poisoning is liver failure. By monitoring serum liver enzymes and performing a liver biopsy, the health care provider can determine what, if any, damage to the liver has occurred. The nurse's responsibilities following a liver biopsy are to monitor hourly vital signs and to place the child on his or her right side on a pillow to provide pressure against the biopsy site to prevent bleeding, the major complication associated with liver biopsies.

10. You overhear Mrs. Chan's phone conversation to consider using Chinese herbal remedies to speed Colman's recovery. Discuss the importance of the nurse's intervention. It is important for the nurse to educate Mrs. Chan that Chinese herbal remedies and other alternative therapies are unlike conventional drugs for which the pharmacodynamics, pharmacokinetics, contraindications, pharmacological side/adverse effects, and their interactive effects with other conventional drugs are clearly defined. Conventional drugs are developed through years of clinical research, trials, and studies as opposed to their alternatives, making it very difficult to determine or predict the consequences of herb–drug interactions.

According to Anna L. Kim, there are currently no regulations designed specifically for herbal medications in the United States. Under current Food and Drug Administration (FDA) procedure, herbal medications may fall within the following regulatory categories: as food, food additives, dietary supplements, or drugs. Herbal medications generally come under the provisions for nutritional supplements because it is difficult for herbal medications to meet the FDA's stringent drug standards and they do not conform exactly to the definitions of food or food additives. Guy Gugliotta of the Washington Post further adds that unlike pharmaceuticals or food additives, supplements do not have to be prescreened by the FDA, nor do they have to demonstrate through peer-reviewed science that they are safe before they can be sold. Once these products are open to public purchase, the burden of proof is on the FDA to show that a supplement is dangerous before it can be taken off the market. Alternative herbal therapies are not FDA regulated today.

A report by the Medicines Control Agency (MCA) in July 2002 indicated that the Agency has continually found traditional Chinese herbals medicines contain potentially dangerous and often illegal ingredients that pose a risk to public health. A survey conducted by MCA on Traditional Chinese Medicines (TCM) revealed 42 different products were found to contain excessive or toxic levels of heavy metals (mercury, lead, arsenic) while 32 different TCM products were found to contain a combined total of 19 drugs. In total, 93 cases of excessive toxic heavy metals and undeclared drugs (most commonly ephedrine, chlorphenirmine, methyltestosterone, and phenacetin) were detected. Other serious quality control related safety problems include lack of, inadequate, or absent labeling of ingredients, differences between the labeled and actual contents, no dose amount or administration frequency for adults versus children, the deliberate addition of prescription medicines, prohibitive or illegal ingredients, toxic heavy metals, and no warnings of intrinsic toxic constituents.

Herbal remedies have traditionally been used by Asian Americans to treat both adults and children. According to Guy Gugliotta, the FDA's monitoring system revealed 2,621 adverse events between 1993 and Oct. 10, 1998,

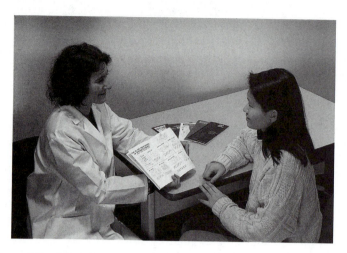

Figure 1-1 *It is important to involve parents in the teaching-learning process.*

with 184 resulting in death. In contrast, The American Association of Poison Control Centers received 6,914 reports on supplements in 1998 alone, including 1,369 cases involving treatment in a health care facility. This figure does not include ephedra and its derivatives. We must also consider that these figures represent only the ones that are reported, as many may have gone unreported. Children are increasingly becoming the victims, with 64% of the association's reports involving children under age 6, a trend also noted among many member poison centers. Pharmacologist Candy Tsououunis at the University of California concurs with these pediatric statistics and added that many supplement bottles or containers tend not to have child-proof caps or seals and supplement companies are providing entire product lines aimed at children that, like their adult equivalents, have not been tested for efficacy, possible side effects, or effects on the young.

Unfortunately, the most common public perception of alternative therapies, specifically herbals, is that they are natural and therefore safer, and the government wouldn't allow unsafe products to be sold. This is why it is imperative for nurses to understand the potential risks posed by the use of alternative therapies and educate clients and their caretakers.

11. Colman recovers and is to be discharged this morning. Discuss the teaching priorities for Colman's parents.

    a. Assess Mr. and Mrs. Chan's current level of understanding concerning Colman's condition. Provide verbal and written instruction (Fig 1-1) regarding:

        (1) Colman's growth and development and how it places him at risk for injury

    (2) Proper storage of toxic substances, including all medications, in locked cabinets

    (3) Importance of storing substances in their original containers, never repackaging them

    (4) Buying products with child-proof caps

    (5) Teaching children about poison safety

    (6) Having the telephone number of the Poison Control Center beside the telephone

    (7) Importance of follow-up care

    (8) The importance of refraining from using Chinese herbal remedies without contacting physician

  b. Provide sufficient time for Mr. and Mrs. Chan to ask questions, referring them as needed.

  c. Document teaching and the Chan's response.

References

American Association of Poison Control Centers. *http://www.aapcc.org*

Centers for Disease Control. *http://www.cdc.gov*

Daniels, R. (2002). *Delmar's manual of laboratory and diagnostic tests.* Clifton Park, NY: Thomson Delmar Learning.

Farrell, S.E. (2004). Toxicity, Acetaminophen. *http://www.emedicine.com*

Gugliotta, G. (2000, March 19). Herbal products take a human toll. Alternative medicines promise health, but often don't deliver. *Washington Post.* Retrieved January 22, 2005.

http://www.fhma.com/herbal_products.htm

Kim, A.L. (1997, May 1). Searching for a Cure: The FDA's Regulatory Approach to Traditional Chinese Herbal Medicine. Submitted to Professor Peter Barton Hutt in the Seminar on Food and Drug Law in Satisfaction of the Written Work Requirement. Retrieved January 21, 2005.

http://leda.law.harvard.edu/leda/data/187/akim.pdf

Medicines Control Agency. (July 2002). Safety of Herbal Medicinal Products. Retrieved January 21, 2005. *http://www.mca.gov.uk/ourwork/licensingmeds/herbalsSafetyReportJuly2002_Final.pdf*

North American Nursing Diagnosis Association. (2005). *Nursing diagnoses: Definitions & classifications, 2005–2006.* Philadelphia: NANDA.

Potts, N. and Mandleco, B. (2002). *Pediatric nursing: Caring for children and their families.* Clifton Park, NY: Thomson Delmar Learning, pp. 685–688.

Spratto, G.R. and Woods, A.L. (2005). *2005 Edition: PDR nurse's drug handbook.* Clifton Park, NY: Thomson Delmar Learning.

Wong, D.L., Perry, S.E., and Hockenberry, M.J. (2002). *Maternal child nursing care* (2nd ed.). St. Louis: Mosby, pp. 1295–1304.

Juan

GENDER

M

AGE

5

SETTING

- Hospital

ETHNICITY

- Spanish American

CULTURAL CONSIDERATIONS

- Hispanic

PREEXISTING CONDITIONS

COEXISTING CONDITIONS

COMMUNICATION

- Spanish-speaking with limited English

DISABILITY

SOCIOECONOMIC

- Middle class

SPIRITUAL

PHARMACOLOGIC

- Cefazolin sodium (Ancet)
- Morphine sulfate (Duramorph)
- Acetominophen (Tylenol)
- Ondansetron hydrochloride (Zofran)

PSYCHOSOCIAL

- Parental anxiety
- Language barrier

LEGAL

ETHICAL

ALTERNATIVE THERAPY

PRIORITIZATION

DELEGATION

- Support staff

MODERATE

THE DIGESTIVE SYSTEM

Level of difficulty: Moderate

Overview: This case requires knowledge of appendicitis, the impact of growth and development on care, the importance of communication, as well as an understanding of the client's background and personal situation.

Client Profile

Juan Sanchez is a 5-year-old preschooler who lives on a farm with his parents, who work as migrant laborers. He is the youngest of four children and the family is a very close-knit family unit. As they recently moved to the United States from Mexico, Spanish is their primary language. His mother neither speaks nor understands English; however, his older brothers and sister can communicate in English that they have learned attending the local school. Juan is a normal preschooler who enjoys playing with his cousins (who live next door) and his siblings after they return from school each day. He does not attend preschool and was never in daycare as his mother stays at home with the children.

Case Study

You receive Juan on the pediatric surgical unit from the emergency department to which his mother brought him with nausea and vomiting. He is crying and guarding the lower right quadrant of his abdomen. His transfer vital signs are:

Temperature: 38.5° C (101.3° F)
Pulse: 110 beats/minute
Respirations: 28 breaths/minute
Blood pressure: 128/78

and he vomits twice during the admission assessment. He had 200 mL of dark green emesis. The transfer nurse reports to you that Juan had an abdominal ultrasound, complete blood count was drawn, and urinalysis was sent to the lab for culture and sensitivity in the emergency department, that neither Juan nor his mother speaks or understands English, and that his father, who does speak English, is on his way to the hospital but has not arrived yet.

Questions

1. Discuss your impressions about the above situation.

2. What additional information would be helpful as you plan Juan's care?

3. Compare the pathophysiology and clinical manifestations of appendicitis and urinary tract infection.

4. Juan's mother is noticeable upset and confused as you examine Juan. How can you help her understand what is going on and decrease her anxiety level?

5. Juan's transfer prescriptions are as follows:

Admission diagnosis: Rule out appendicitis versus urinary tract infection
5% Dextrose and 0.2% normal saline intravenous fluids to infuse at 90 mL/hour
Cefazolin sodium 450 mg IV now
Morphine sulfate 2 mg IV every 1–2 hours PRN pain
Ondansetron hydrochloride 2 mg IV now

Questions (continued)

Acetaminophen 120 mg PR every 4 hours for temperature >38° (100.4° F)
Nothing by mouth.
How do you explain what the health care provider has prescribed for Juan?

6. You find that one of the housekeepers on the unit speaks Spanish and you recruit him to communicate with Juan and his mother. What information should you ask to be communicated to them?

7. On admission to your unit, Juan weighed 19 kg (41.8 lb). Are the dosages prescribed safe for Juan?

8. After you medicate Juan with morphine sulfate, he remains alert but tells his mother that the pain is much better since she put the warm towel on his tummy. This is translated to you. What is your impression concerning Juan's response?

9. Forty-five minutes after you medicate Juan with the morphine sulfate, the acetaminophen for his fever, and his first dose of cefazolin sodium, Juan's temperature is 39° C (102.2° F) and he has become nonresponsive. His pulse rate is 126 beats/minute, his respirations are 36 per minute, and his blood pressure is 130/80. What is your impression of this data and what immediate actions should you take?

10. Juan's father has not arrived at the hospital yet and even with explanations,

Juan's mother is reluctant to sign the informed consent until her husband arrives. As Juan is being transferred to surgery, his father arrives and after the health care provider's explanation, he signs the consent and Juan is rushed into surgery where an emergency appendectomy is performed for a ruptured appendix. He returns to the pediatric surgical floor following 2 hours in the post-anesthesia care unit post-anesthesia care unit (PACU) with the following medical prescriptions:

- Salem sump nasogastric tube to low intermittent wall suction
- Routine vital signs
- 5% Dextrose and 0.2% normal saline intravenous fluids to infuse at 90 mL/hour
- Cefazolin sodium 500 mg IV now
- Morphine sulfate 2 mg IV every 1–2 hours PRN pain
- Acetaminophen 240 mg PR every 4 hours for temperature >38° C (100.4° F)
- Nothing by mouth
- Strict intake and output
- OOB (out of bed) in the morning
- Call House Officer if temperature is greater than 38.4° C (101° F)

Discuss the nursing responsibilities when caring for a client with a nasogastric tube to low intermittent wall suction.

Questions and Suggested Answers

1. Discuss your impressions about the above situation. The clinical manifestations point to appendicitis and perhaps a urinary tract infection (UTI). The cardinal manifestations of appendicitis are generalized abdominal pain radiating to the right lower quadrant where the appendix is located, nausea and vomiting, and fever. Juan has all of these manifestations. Although rare in children younger than 4 years of age, appendicitis leading to an appendectomy occurs in 4 of 1,000 children older than the age of 4. Urinary tract infections are much more common in very young girls because of the closer structural relationship between the urethra and the anus in girls; however,

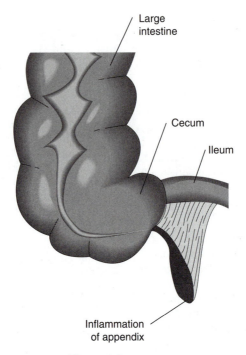

Large intestine

Cecum

Ileum

Inflammation of appendix

Figure 1-2   *Appendix.*

among Spanish-speaking individuals cultural conventions prescribe that infant males should not be circumcised, which would increase Juan's chances of urinary tract infections. The cardinal manifestations of urinary tract infections are urgency, burning, and frequency of urination and the scenario does not address these symptoms. The fact that neither he nor his mother speak or understand English will create a challenge for nurses.

2.   What additional information would be helpful as you plan Juan's care? How old are Juan's siblings? Would his older siblings be able to assist the nurse in communicating with Juan's mother? What are the results of Juan's abdominal ultrasound? Has informed consent been signed for Juan's surgery? What is Juan's weight? What are the results of his complete blood count (CBC), urinalysis (UA), and culture and sensitivity (C&S)?

3.   Compare the pathophysiology and clinical manifestations of appendicitis and urinary tract infection. APPENDICITIS: The appendix normally fills with digested food and empties into the cecum (Fig. 1-2). When this normal emptying does not occur, the appendix can become obstructed by intestinal contents (including intestinal microbial flora) and an accumulation of mucous secretions. This results in distention of the appendix that leads to engorgement of the veins and capillaries that supply the appendix with blood. The increased pressure within the lumen compromises vascular supply. This can lead to small abscesses, necrosis, and eventual perforation of the intestinal wall or the pressure can exceed what the wall of the appendix can tolerate and the appendix ruptures. Whether perforation or rupture occurs, the bacteria from the intestines leak into the peritoneal cavity, resulting in peritonitis. Appendicitis is manifested by generalized abdominal pain radiating to the lower right quadrant where the appendix is located, fever, and nausea and vomiting. The cardinal symptom of appendix rupture is a sudden relief of the abdominal pain followed by a deterioration in the client's condition as peritonitis progresses. If untreated, this will lead to sepsis.

URINARY TRACT INFECTION: Under the right conditions, bacteria from the intestines present in feces is transported to the urinary meatus by poor hygiene practices, such as wiping from back to front after a bowel movement; underwear that is worn too tight; improper bladder emptying; and contamination from bath water (the urethra dilates when it comes in contact with warm liquids, thus allowing bacteria in bath water to travel up the urethra to the urinary bladder). Once the intestinal bacteria enter the sterile urinary system, bacterial growth increases, causing irritation and infection in the urinary system. The cardinal manifestations of a UTI are urgency, frequency, and burning on urination. Children also may be febrile.

4. Juan's mother is noticeably upset and confused as you examine Juan. How can your approach help her understand what is going on and decrease her anxiety level? Assess whether there is another staff member who speaks Spanish. Contact the hospital's Spanish interpreter, if available. Use nonverbal communication, such as hand gestures and demonstrations of what the nurse is doing. Owing to the dramatic increase in the Spanish-speaking population in the United States today (they are the largest minority population), many health care facilities, especially state university-based hospitals and those with large numbers of admissions of Spanish-speaking individuals, have resources to assist nursing in communicating with this population. For example, reference books, pamphlets, interpreters, etc. address this health issue. In addition, faculties of nursing programs are increasingly encouraging their nursing students to learn Spanish as a second language. Although it would not help this situation, taking one to two courses in Spanish by the practicing nurse as continuing education would be beneficial to both the nurse and to future Spanish-speaking clients and their families.

5. Juan's transfer prescriptions are as follows:
Admission diagnosis: Rule out appendicitis versus urinary tract infection
5% Dextrose and 0.2% normal saline intravenous fluids to infuse at 90 mL/hour
Cefazolin sodium 500 mg IV now
Morphine sulfate 2 mg IV every 1–2 hours PRN pain

Ondansetron hydrochloride 2 mg IV now
Acetaminophen 240 mg PR every 4 hours for temperature >38° C (100.4° F)
Nothing by mouth
Strict intake and output

How do you explain what the health care provider has prescribed for Juan? The intravenous fluids are used to increase Juan's fluid intake and replace fluids lost during vomiting. This is necessary because of the fragile nature of fluid and electrolyte balance in children. The intravenous access also provides a route for Juan's medications. Cefazolin sodium is a semisynthetic, first-generation, broad-spectrum cephalosporin that is used to treat infections of the GI tract and prior to surgeries of the GI and GU systems as prophylaxis. Morphine sulfate is a potent opioid narcotic that is the drug of choice for moderate to severe pain in children. A side effect of morphine is slowing of bowel motility that may decrease the risk of Juan's appendix rupturing. Ondansetron hydrochloride is a potent antiemetic that acts by blocking serotonin. Acetaminophen is a non-narcotic analgesic and effective antipyretic. Because children are at risk for febrile seizures, acetaminophen is used to decrease the body temperature. The NPO status has three purposes: (1) to decrease stomach contents that pose a risk of aspiration for clients experiencing vomiting, (2) to decrease intestinal motility, and (3) prior to administering systemic anesthesia in surgery, the client should have no oral intake for a minimum of 4 hours to prevent nausea and vomiting sometimes associated with general anesthesia. Strict intake and output is used to measure Juan's fluid balance and monitor for the effectiveness of fluid resuscitation.

6. You find that one of the housekeepers on the unit speaks Spanish and you recruit him to communicate with Juan and his mother. What information should you ask to be communicated to them? Juan's mother needs a simple explanation of Juan's condition. This can be conveyed to her by a nonprofessional by explaining that Juan has an infection in his intestines. If the mother does not understand the word intestines, she can be told that it is an infection in Juan's stomach. Explaining that the intravenous fluids are "going into Juan to replace the fluids he lost as a result of his vomiting (throwing up). Further, she can be told that the nurse is listening to Juan's heart, lungs, stomach, etc. to "make sure he is OK." The medications should be explained simply in terms of why Juan is receiving them. Prior to administration of any drug, the nurse needs to determine whether Juan has any drug allergies. The most important concept in this teaching is simplicity not only for the nonprofessional doing the interpreting, but also for Juan's mother who is obviously anxious about her son's condition and in the presence of anxiety, complicated explanations can easily lead to misunderstanding. The use of nonprofessional personnel is not recommended because of confidentiality and potential legal risks, however, if a Spanish-speaking professional is not available and only simple information is conveyed through the non-professional, this may be necessary in limited cases.

7. On admission to your unit, Juan weighed 41.8 lb. Are the dosages prescribed safe for Juan? The safe dosage for cefazolin sodium is 8.3 to 33.3 mg/kg of body weight every 8 hours. Juan's safe range is 157.7 to 632.7 mg every 8 hours, so his dose of the drug is safe. The safe dosage range for morphine sulfate is 0.1–0.2 mg/kg per dose. Juan can receive between 1.9 and 3.8 mg/dose so the prescribed dose of morphine sulfate for Juan is safe. The safe dosage range for ondansetron hydrochloride is 0.1 mg–0.15 mg/kg per dose. Juan can receive 1.9 to 2.85 mg of ondansetron per dose. His dose is 2 mg is safe. The safe dosage range for acetaminophen is 10 to 15 mg/kg per dose so Juan can receive up to 285 mg/dose based on his weight. All of Juan's prescribed doses are safe.

8. After you medicate Juan with morphine sulfate, he remains alert but tells his mother that the pain is much better since she put the warm towel on his "tummy." This is translated to you. What is your impression concerning Juan's response? Although the nurse's first impression may be that the morphine sulfate has been effective in controlling Juan's pain, another consideration should be that the cardinal sign of appendix rupture is sudden relief of pain. In addition, applying any source of heat to the abdomen of a client suspected of appendicitis is contraindicated because the heat dilates blood vessels and can increase the pressure within the appendix increasing the risk of rupture. Juan should be closely monitored and the health care provider informed.

9. Forty-five minutes after you medicate Juan with the morphine sulfate, the acetaminophen for his fever, and his first dose of cefazolin sodium, Juan's temperature is 39° C (102.2° F) and he has become nonresponsive. His pulse rate is 126 beats/minute, his respirations are 36 breaths/minute, and his blood pressure is 130/80. What is your impression of this data and what immediate actions should you take? Juan's vital signs and his sudden relief of pain are indications of appendix rupture. The nurse needs to immediately notify his health care provider and prepare Juan for emergency surgery. As the nurse prepares Juan, he/she must remain calm and have the interpreter explain to his mother in simple terms the reason for the rush of preparation activities. The health care provider may prescribe a stat abdominal ultrasound and prepare him for transfer to the ultrasound department.

10. Juan's father has not arrived at the hospital yet and even with explanations, Juan's mother is reluctant to sign the informed consent until her husband arrives. As Juan is being transferred to surgery, his father arrives and after the health care provider's explanation, he signs the consent and

Juan is rushed into surgery where an emergency appendectomy is performed for a ruptured appendix. He returns to the pediatric surgical floor following 2 hours in PACU with the following medical prescriptions:
Salem sump nasogastric tube to low intermittent wall suction
Routine vital signs
5% Dextrose and 0.2% normal saline intravenous fluids to infuse at 90 mL/hour
Cefazolin sodium 500 mg IV now
Morphine sulfate 2 mg IV every 1–2 hours PRN pain
Acetaminophen 240 mg PR every 4 hours for temperature >38° C (100.4° F)
Nothing by mouth
Strict intake and output
Out of bed (OOB) in the morning
Call House Officer if temperature is greater than 38.4° C (101° F)

Discuss the nursing responsibilities when caring for a client with a nasogastric tube to low intermittent wall suction. The nurse's first responsibility is to check the facility procedure for the care and maintenance of nasogastric (NG) tubes. This discussion will address the standards of care. The nurse needs to have the equipment ready including a wall suction meter, drainage canister, drainage tubing, and tubing to attach the canister to the wall suction meter. Sterile normal saline for irrigation and a sterile irrigation set including a 30- to 60-mL syringe and an irrigation receptacle should be at the client's bedside. Prior to attaching the NG tube to suction, the nurse should check the tube for proper placement by instilling 5 mL of air into the NG tube while auscultating over the epigastric area with a stethoscope. Following verification of proper placement, the nurse should attach the NG tube to the suction tubing and set the suction meter for 20 cm (7.9 in.) of intermittent suction. The Salem sump NG tube has holes in the end of it (the end in the stomach) for the drainage to be suctioned through and an air vent at the other end where the tube is attached to the suction tubing. When attached to wall suction, a "whistling" sound (from air passing through the air vent) should be audible from the end of the air vent. If this doesn't occur, the nurse should instill 5 mL of air into the air vent.

NOTE: The air vent has a seal where it attaches to the NG tube and only air should be instilled into the air vent. Any other substance including normal saline will break the seal if it is instilled into the air vent and the system will not function properly. Instilling the small amount of air should clear the tube and drainage should begin to flow through the NG tube and into the suction canister as the air vent whistles. If this does not work, the nurse should reposition the client as the NG tube may be too close to the gastric wall which can prohibit drainage from entering the tube. If drainage is still not coming through the tube, the nurse should irrigate the NG tube gently with 5–10 mL of sterile normal saline for irrigation to clear the tube of drainage that may be blocking it. Further, the nurse is responsible for keeping strict intake and output records of the NG drainage and document this information. In situations in which excessive NG drainage occurs or is anticipated or with clients whose fluid and electrolyte balance is fragile the health care provider may prescribe that the NG drainage volume be replaced by intravenous fluids. In children, the replacement is usually done every 2–4 hours to avoid large replacement volumes needing to be replaced at the end of the shift which could compromise the IV access.

References

Broyles, B.E. (2005). *Medical-surgical nursing clinical companion.* Durham, NC: Carolina Academic Press.

Centers for Disease Control. *http://www.cdc.gov*

Daniels, R. (2002). *Delmar's manual of laboratory and diagnostic tests.* Clifton Park, NY: Thomson Delmar Learning.

Gahart, B.L. and Nazareno, A.R. (2005). *2005 Intravenous medications* (21st ed.). St. Louis: Mosby.

Intravenous Therapy. *http://www.nursewise.com*

North American Nursing Diagnosis Association. (2005). *Nursing diagnoses: Definitions & classifications, 2005–2006.* Philadelphia: NANDA.

Potts, N. and Mandleco, B. (2002). *Pediatric nursing: Caring for children and their families.* Clifton Park, NY: Thomson Delmar Learning.

Wong, D.L., Perry, S.E., and Hockenberry, M.J. (2002). *Maternal child nursing care* (2nd ed.). St. Louis: Mosby, pp. 1268–1269.

Daniel

GENDER

M

AGE

13 months old

SETTING

- Hospital

ETHNICITY

- White American

CULTURAL CONSIDERATIONS

PREEXISTING CONDITIONS

- Biliary atresia

COEXISTING CONDITIONS

COMMUNICATION

DISABILITY

SOCIOECONOMIC

SPIRITUAL

PHARMACOLOGIC

- Cyclosporine (Restasis)
- Tacrolimus (Prograf)
- Azathioprine (Imuran)

PSYCHOSOCIAL

- Divorced parents

LEGAL

ETHICAL

ALTERNATIVE THERAPY

PRIORITIZATION

DELEGATION

DIFFICULT

THE DIGESTIVE SYSTEM

Level of difficulty: Difficult

Overview: This case requires knowledge of biliary atresia and understanding of the client's background, personal situation, and how these may affect parent–child interaction.

Client Profile

Daniel is a 13-month-old who lives with his mother; his 7-year-old brother, Jon; and his 4-year-old sister, Valerie. Daniel weighed 3.4 kg (7.5 lb) at birth. When Daniel was 4 weeks old he developed jaundice and an enlarged abdomen. After diagnostic tests were completed, he was diagnosed with biliary atresia. At 8 weeks of age, he underwent a successful Kasai procedure. Daniel's condition placed a strain on his parent's marriage and they were divorced 4 months ago. His father takes his brother and sister every other weekend and interacts briefly with Daniel when he comes to pick up Jon and Valerie. His father provides sufficient child support and insurance to pay Daniel's medical bills. His alimony payments allow Daniel's mother to stay at home and care for Daniel. She also works part-time from her home to supplement the family income.

Case Study

Daniel weighs 6.8 kg (15 lb) and over the past year he has experienced recurrent episodes of ascending cholangitis. Over the past 6 weeks, Daniel has developed ascites that did not respond to conservative treatment and has episodes of variceal bleeding. His current platelet count is 15, 000 cells/mm^3, and his vital signs are:

Temperature: 35° C (95° F)
Pulse: 120 beats/minute
Respirations: 35 breaths/minute
Blood pressure: 95/50

His liver enzymes are below the normal range, and his urinalysis indicates bilirubin in his urine.

Questions

1. Discuss your impressions of Daniel's father's reaction to Daniel's condition.

2. What is biliary atresia?

3. What is the Kasai procedure and how is it used to help children with biliary atresia?

4. Discuss the significance of Daniel's current clinical manifestations.

5. What is the relationship between Daniel's laboratory values and his diagnosis?

6. Daniel is experiencing liver failure. Discuss the complications of this condition.

7. The transplant team discusses with Daniel's mother and father Daniel's need for a liver transplant. Both of his parents volunteer to be the donor. Discuss your impression of Daniel's father's response to Daniel's need for a transplant, identifying any biases you may have.

8. Discuss live donor liver transplants and their use in children with liver failure.

Questions (continued)

9. Daniel's mother asks the nursing staff how common liver transplants are and what their success rates are as she considers Daniel's risks. How would you respond to her concerns?

10. Identify the complications associated with Daniel receiving a transplanted liver.

11. Daniel's mother is determined to be a genetic match for Daniel. How is the donor liver processed prior to transplant?

12. Daniel receives part of his mother's liver. What are the priorities of care for Daniel following his transplant?

13. Discuss the nursing interventions needed to meet Daniel's care needs.

14. Daniel is recovering from his transplant and his transplant physician prescribes cyclosporine 25 mg PO b.i.d., tacrolimus 1 mg PO b.i.d., and azathioprine 14 mg PO every day. Discuss this medication regimen and how it relates to Daniel's transplant.

15. Would you question any of the doses prescribed for Daniel?

Questions and Suggested Answers

1.   Discuss your impressions of Daniel's father's reaction to Daniel's condition. Grief is a common reaction among parents who have a child with a chronic and potentially life-threatening illness. The first step in the grief process is denial and the second is anger. Daniel's father may not have been able to move past these first steps, preventing him from moving to the point of acceptance. All infants bring with them some degree of stress into the family unit; those that have a chronic condition unintentionally increase that stress. He was unable to develop a loving relationship with Daniel, but his financial contributions indicate that he accepts the responsibility for Daniel. His relationship with Jon appears strong and may eventually help him accept Daniel.

2.   What is biliary atresia? Biliary atresia or extrahepatic biliary atresia (EHBA) is the congenital absence or obstruction of the bile ducts. This results in inflammation that leads to intrahepatic and extrahepatic bile duct fibrosis. Eventually, the backup of bile in the liver leads to liver failure. The cause is unknown. It occurs slightly more often in girls than boys and has an incidence of 1:10,000 to 1:25,000 live births.

3.   What is the Kasai procedure and how is it used the help children with biliary atresia? According to the American Liver Foundation, the Kasai procedure, when performed before the infant is 10 weeks old, achieves bile drainage in 80% to 90% of cases of biliary atresia. During the procedure, "the surgeon removes the damaged ducts outside of the liver (extrahepatic) and replaces them with a length of the baby's own intestine, which acts as a new duct" that allows bile to drain into the gall bladder and then into the duodenum of the small intestines. In those who respond well to the procedure, jaundice is resolved within a few weeks. This procedure corrects the extrahepatic but not the intrahepatic duct obstruction, which eventually requires a liver transplant.

4. Discuss the significance of Daniel's current clinical manifestations. Daniel's current clinical manifestations indicate that his liver is failing. These symptoms are indications of a need for a liver transplant. Daniel weighed 3.4 kg or 7 lb 8 oz at birth and infants normally triple their weight in the first year of life. Daniel's current weight is only twice his birth weight. This is evidence of growth failure. He experienced recurrent episodes of ascending cholangitis, and during the past 6 weeks, he has developed ascites that did not respond to conservative treatment. He also has experienced episodes of variceal bleeding. These are indicators of the need for a liver transplant. His vital signs indicate tachycardia and tachypnea, both indicators of ineffective tissue perfusion that the heart and lungs are attempting to compensate. The hypoperfusion is related to anemia that occurs in the presence of liver failure. His tachypnea also may be the result of ascites that occurs when the liver cannot function. Ascites places pressure against the diaphragm that interferes with lung compliance and vital capacity. His temperature is below normal, which occurs with the loss of body heat when the liver cannot perform its chemical and metabolic functions.

5. What is the relationship between Daniel's laboratory values and his diagnosis? Daniel's current platelet count of 15, 000 cells/mm^3 indicates thrombocytopenia resulting from increased activity of the spleen that occurs when the liver is failing. This also is an indicator of the need for a liver transplant in a child with biliary atresia. More than 70% of the parenchymal cells in the liver may be damaged before any changes in the liver enzymes occur. That Daniel's enzymes are below the normal range probably indicates a substantial loss of the parenchyma. Bilirubin in the urine also indicates impairment of liver function.

6. Daniel is experiencing liver failure. Discuss the complications of this condition. The complications associated with liver failure are directly correlated to the loss of multiple functions of the liver. Altered coagulation that leads to thrombocytopenia and bleeding result from the liver's inability to synthesize prothrombin and fibrinogen and manufacture heparin. With the inability to metabolize and detoxify chemicals (including drugs), toxic levels of medications occur. The liver normally synthesizes almost all of the plasma proteins necessary to maintain vascular osmotic pressure. When the liver fails, there is decreased serum albumin with resulting edema and ascites. The liver normally breaks down red blood cells into bilirubin; when it can no longer perform this function, jaundice occurs with resulting pruritus. The liver has a major responsibility in gastrointestinal function including the manufacture and release of bile necessary for fat digestion and metabolism, storage for large amounts of vitamins including A, B_{12}, D, and other B complex vitamins; metabolism of carbohydrates and proteins; regulation of blood sugar by converting glucose to glycogen for storage and then converting it back to glucose as needed for energy; synthesis of glucose using amino acids from protein metabolism; and synthesis of protein resulting in the formation of ammonia for excretion as urea. The elevated ammonia levels lead to hepatic encephalopathy and eventually hepatic coma. In the presence of liver failure, the child experiences malabsorption, vitamin deficiencies, hyperglycemia from the inability to convert glucose to stored glycogen, and hypoglycemia from lack of glycogen stores. The healthy liver produces heat for the body from the many chemical reactions it performs. The child with liver failure experiences decreased body temperature that can progress to hypothermia. Anemia is another complication of liver failure.

7. **The transplant team discusses with Daniel's mother and father Daniel's need for a liver transplant. Both of his parents volunteer to be the donor. Discuss your impression of Daniel's father's response to Daniel's need for a transplant, identifying any biases you may have.** Daniel's father may be progressing through his initial grief response and has moved to acceptance of Daniel and his need for a compatible donor. Some readers may have negative feelings about the father including the need to punish him for abandoning his family after Daniel's birth and diagnosis. This is not the appropriate focus for the nurse. The major concern should be Daniel and what is best for him. What he needs most now is a genetically compatible donor and both his parents are willing to be tested for compatibility and to be his donor if possible.

8. **Discuss live donor liver transplants and their use in children with liver failure.** The first live donor liver transplant on a child was performed in 1989. According to 2003 annual report of the U.S. Organ Procurement and Transplantation Network, "In 2002, 72 children received living donor liver transplants, accounting for 20% of all living donor liver transplant recipients. Children aged 5 years and younger accounted for 86% of pediatric living donor liver recipients." When the liver donor is the child's parent, immunologic benefits may occur, decreasing the incidence of rejection. Live donor liver transplants have a reported recipient survival of 85% and a graft survival of 75%. Because 80% of children needing liver transplants are under the age of 2 years and the difficulty in finding appropriately sized cadaver livers, reduced-sized liver transplantation was developed.

9. Daniel's mother asks the nursing staff how common liver transplants are and their success rate as she considers Daniel's risks. How would you respond to her concerns? According to the U.S. Organ Procurement and Transplantation Network and the United Network for Organ Sharing, since 1988 more than 3,200 liver transplants were performed on children between the ages of 1 and 5 years. In 2002, these children had a 1-year survival rate of 85–95% and 3-year and 5-year survival rates of approximately 84%. The leading cause of mortality for any type of transplant is infection secondary to immunosuppressant therapy needed to prevent organ rejection.

10. Identify the complications associated with Daniel receiving a transplanted liver.

    a. Acute graft rejection leading to possible need for retransplantation

    b. Life-threatening infections secondary to immunosuppressant therapy

    c. Posttransplant lymphoproliferative disorder associated with immunosuppressant therapy

    d. Hemorrhage

    e. Hepatic artery thrombosis

    f. Fluid and electrolyte imbalances

    g. Pulmonary atelectasis

    h. Nephrotoxicity related to the use of cyclosporine

11. Daniel's mother is determined to be a genetic match for Daniel. How is the donor liver processed prior to transplant? With live donor liver transplants the left lateral lobe of the liver is resected and the donor liver is then flushed with cold lactated Ringer's solution to remove potassium and air bubbles.

12. Daniel receives part of his mother's liver. What are the priorities of care for Daniel following his transplant?

    a. Impaired gas exchange related to atelectasis secondary to surgical approach

    b. Acute pain related to surgical incision and presence of chest tubes

    c. High risk for infection related to immunosuppressant state, surgical incision, invasive tubes

    d. Risk for injury, organ rejection related to body's immune response to reject foreign matter

    e. Risk for injury, bleeding related to altered coagulation ability

    f. Risk injury, complications secondary to liver transplantation related to cardiovascular, renal, neurological, and metabolic functioning

    g. Deficient knowledge (parental) related to transplant, post-operative course, and home care

13. Discuss the nursing interventions needed to meet Daniel's care needs.

a. Gas exchange
  (1) Monitor respiratory status continuously.
  (2) Monitor pulmonary capillary wedge pressure.
  (3) Monitor serial arterial blood gases and pulse oximetry.
  (4) Administer oxygen, titrating to prescribed parameters.
  (5) Maintain closed chest tube drainage system.
  (6) Assist with chest x-ray films as needed to determine readiness to discontinue chest tubes.
  (7) Assist with removal of chest tubes after confirmation of resolved atelectasis.

b. Acute pain
  (1) Assess pain level hourly and as needed including monitoring for nonverbal indicators while Daniel is on mechanical ventilation.
  (2) When Daniel is able to verbalize, assess pain based on verbalization and appropriate pediatric pain assessment tool, such as the combined faces–numerical scale.
  (3) Maintain patency of intravenous access, monitoring hourly.
  (4) Monitor vital signs.
  (5) Monitor continuous intravenous opioid analgesia.
  (6) Place Daniel on continuous cardiorespiratory monitoring and pulse oximetry while he is receiving parenteral opioid analgesia.
  (7) Be proactive in pain management.
  (8) Position for comfort.

c. Infection
  (1) Monitor body temperature continuously with skin probe according to critical care protocol.
  (2) Monitor body temperature every 4 hours following the acute postoperative period.
  (3) Monitor for wound, tube, and line drainage.
  (4) Obtain cultures as prescribed.
  (5) Monitor complete blood count with differential.
  (6) Maintain patency of intravenous access, monitoring hourly and as needed.
  (7) Administer antibiotics as prescribed if infection occurs.
  (8) Collaborate with the health care provider to remove invasive lines and tubes as early as possible.
  (9) Perform handwashing according to the transplant protocol.
  (10) Instruct family and visitors about proper handwashing techniques

d. Organ rejection
  (1) Assess for signs and symptoms of liver failure.
  (2) Monitor liver function tests.

      (3) Monitor for increasing jaundice, presence of tachycardia, and other manifestations of rejection.

      (4) Administer immunosuppressant agents as prescribed.

      (5) Monitor of adverse effect of immunosuppressant therapy (nephrotoxicity)

e. Bleeding

      (1) Monitor for bleeding from wound, T-tube, chest tubes.

      (2) Monitor complete blood count.

      (3) Test urine for blood.

      (4) Hemoccult stools.

      (5) Place Daniel on Bleeding Precautions.

      (6) Monitor coagulation studies and report abnormalities immediately.

f. Complications

      (1) Monitor cardiovascular status including cardiac output, central venous pressure, heart rate, blood pressure, electrocardiography.

      (2) Monitor pulmonary function including pulmonary capillary wedge pressure, arterial blood gases venous blood gases, chest tube drainage, mechanical ventilation settings.

      (3) Monitor renal function including urinary output, arterial blood gases, blood urea nitrogen (BUN), creatinine, and blood pressure.

      (4) Monitor neurological functioning.

      (5) Monitor metabolic functioning including liver function tests, electrolyte levels, coagulation studies, biliary drainage

      (6) Report abnormal findings (outside prescribed parameters) immediately

g. Parental teaching

      (1) Encourage parental visiting.

      (2) Assess parents' current level of knowledge.

      (3) Explain all medications, equipment, and procedures.

      (4) Prior to Daniel's discharge, provide verbal and written information regarding:

         (a) Risk factors for developing infection and signs and symptoms (temperature elevations >37.8° C [100° F]) to report immediately to the health care provider

         (b) Signs and symptoms of rejection and importance of reporting them immediately to health care provider

         (c) Medication administration including importance of compliance with prescribed medication regimen

(d) Signs and symptoms of adverse effects of medications (decreased renal function)

(e) Dressing changes, if needed

(f) Signs and symptoms of worsening of condition

(g) Contact phone numbers to report signs and symptoms

(h) Importance of regular handwashing and appropriate technique

(i) Importance of immediate and long-term follow-up with health care provider

(5) Always provide for sufficient time for client and family questions, answering them honestly.

(6) Document teaching and client and family response

14. Daniel is recovering from his transplant and his transplant physician prescribes cyclosporine 25 mg PO b.i.d., tacrolimus 1 mg PO b.i.d., and azathioprine 14 mg PO every day. Discuss this medication regimen and how it relates to Daniel's transplant. These are immunosuppressant agents used to prevent organ rejection. Another immunosuppressant approved for use in children is muromonab-CD3 (OKT). Corticosteroids are used in conjunction with the immunosuppressant agents.

15. Would you question any of the doses prescribed for Daniel? Daniel weighs 15 lb, or 6.82 kg. The safe dosage range of cyclosporine is 5–10 mg/kg per day so Daniel's safe range is 34.1–68.2 mg each day. Daniel's daily dose is given in divided doses to help prevent the most common adverse effect of cyclosporine, which is nephrotoxicity. The safe dosage range of tacrolimus is 0.15–0.3 mg/kg per day. Daniel can receive 1–2 mg per day. The safe dosage range of azathioprine is 1–3 mg/kg so Daniel can receive 6.82–20.46 mg each day. All of his prescribed doses are safe so the nurse would not question the prescription for these medications. The nurse may collaborate with the transplant team concerning the use of corticosteroids in conjunction with Daniel's immunosuppressants.

References

Centers for Disease Control. *http://www.cdc.gov*

Daniels, R. (2002). *Delmar's manual of laboratory and diagnostic tests.* Clifton Park, NY: Thomson Delmar Learning.

Gahart, B.L. and Nazareno, A.R. (2005). *2005 Intravenous medications* (21st ed.). St. Louis: Mosby.

National Library of Medicine. *http://www.nlm.nih.gov*

North American Nursing Diagnosis Association. (2005). *Nursing diagnoses: Definitions & classifications, 2005–2006.* Philadelphia: NANDA.

Potts, N. and Mandleco, B. (2002). *Pediatric nursing: Caring for children and their families.* Clifton Park, NY: Thomson Delmar Learning, pp. 691–692.

Spratto, G.R. and Woods, A.L. (2005). *2005 Edition: PDR nurse's drug handbook.* Clifton Park, NY: Thomson Delmar Learning.

United Network for Organ Sharing. *http://www.unos.org*

U.S. Organ Procurement and Transplantation Network. *http://www.optn.org*

Wong, D.L., Perry, S.E., and Hockenberry, M.J. (2002). *Maternal child nursing care* (2nd ed.). St. Louis: Mosby, pp. 1278–1279.

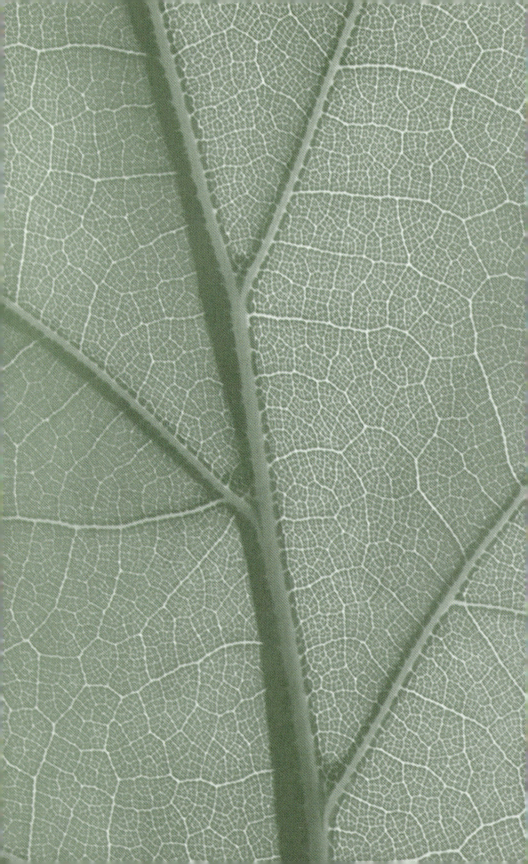

PART TWO

Nasal cavity

Oral cavity
(mouth)

Pharynx
(throat)

Larynx
(voice box)

Trachea
(windpipe)

Bronchus

Lungs

Diaphragm

Respiratory system Lungs,
nasal cavity, pharynx, larynx,
trachea, bronchi, and bronchioles.

The Respiratory System

CASE STUDY 1

Sok Wu

GENDER	**SOCIOECONOMIC**
M	
AGE	**SPIRITUAL**
4	
SETTING	**PHARMACOLOGIC**
■ Emergency room	■ Cetazolin (Ancef)
ETHNICITY	**PSYCHOSOCIAL**
■ Asian American	■ Anxiety
CULTURAL CONSIDERATION	**LEGAL**
PREEXISTING CONDITIONS	**ETHICAL**
COEXISTING CONDITIONS	**ALTERNATIVE THERAPY**
COMMUNICATION	**PRIORITIZATION**
■ English/Chinese	■ Emergency situation
DISABILITY	**DELEGATION**
	■ Nurse assistant
	■ Client teaching

THE RESPIRATORY SYSTEM

Level of difficulty: Easy

Overview: This case requires knowledge of foreign body aspiration (FBA), growth and developmental risks for FBA, as well as an understanding of the client's background, personal situation, and family–child relationship.

Client Profile

Sok Wu Yang is a preschooler who is celebrating his fourth birthday today. He lives with his mother, aunt, siblings, and grandparents. His father was killed in a construction accident when Sok Wu was an infant. He has a 6-year-old sister and an 8-year-old brother. His mother and aunt are fluent in both Chinese and English, although his grandparents speak only Chinese. He and his siblings also are fluent in both languages, speaking their native language when conversing with their grandparents and English with their mother and aunt. Sok Wu, nicknamed Scotty by his family to facilitate his integration into preschool, enjoys preschool and playing with his friends there. The family has been planning a birthday party for Sok Wu and has invited his preschool class to attend as well as one of his sister's friends and his brother's best friend from school. Sok Wu is very excited about the party and wants to help in all of the preparations.

Case Study

Two hours before his party begins, Sok Wu is brought to the emergency department of the hospital located two blocks from his home by his mother and aunt. His mother is very upset and tells the nurse Sok Wu had "swallowed a party balloon" that he found on the table at home. He is in respiratory distress when his mother and aunt bring him to the hospital. As the nurse assesses the client's airway, she asks the nursing assistant to take Sok Wu's vital signs with the following results:

Temperature: 36° C (96.8° F)
Pulse: 140 beats/minute
Blood pressure: 70/40
Respirations: irregular

The child's pulse oximetry reading is 78% on admission. The nurse's assessment reveals barely audible and diminished breath sounds bilaterally; stridor and use of accessory muscles; heart sounds weak and irregular; cool, clammy skin; and decreased responsiveness.

Questions

1. Discuss your impressions about the above situation.

2. What are the nurse's priority interventions as the child enters the emergency department?

3. What is the significance of Sok Wu's vital signs, oxygen saturation reading, and the nurse's assessment findings?

4. What are the nursing priorities for this situation?

5. Discuss how you think Sok Wu's mother and aunt are feeling at this point.

6. The health care provider prescribes the following for Sok Wu:

Order stat chest X-ray.
Initiate PIV of 5% Dextrose and 0.2%

normal saline to infuse at 70 mL/hour. Monitor oxygen saturation via pulse oximetry.
Maintain nothing by mouth (NPO).
Monitor continuous vital signs.

Following the chest X-ray which reveals a foreign body in his trachea, Sok Wu is scheduled for an emergency bronchoscopy. What is the rationale for this procedure in this case?

7. Following the successful bronchoscopy, what assessments should the nurse perform on Sok Wu?

8. The health care provider prescribes cefazolin 160 mg IV q6h × 3 doses with the first dose to be administered stat. You asked the nursing assistant to weigh Sok Wu on the scales on his hospital bed as you communicate the medication order to pharmacy. The nursing assistant reports that Sok Wu weighs 16.5 kg (36.3 lb). Did the nurse act appropriately when she delegated obtaining Sok Wu's weight to the nursing assistant?

9. What process does the nurse use when administering medications to this child?

10. Describe your feelings about this situation considering Sok Wu's level of growth and development.

11. Thirty-six hours following his admission to the hospital, Sok Wu is discharged with no complications associated with his FBA. He is sent home with his mother and aunt. What would be the nurse's focus in discharge teaching for Sok Wu's mother and aunt?

Questions and Suggested Answers

1. **Discuss your impressions about the above situation.** Sok Wu has probably aspirated the balloon and it is blocking his airway. Because balloons are pliable, they are difficult to expel from the airway using the Heimlich maneuver, usually requiring procedural removal. Because of the other information including his vital signs and the fact that he is still conscious, although barely, the blockage may be partial rather than complete.

2. **What are the nurse's priority interventions as the child enters the emergency department?** The nurse's priorities in this situation include assessing the child airway, breathing, and circulation. Depending on these findings, actions must address maintaining a patent airway, effective respirations, and tissue perfusion.

3. **What is the significance of Sok Wu's vital signs, oxygen saturation, and the nurse's assessment findings?** The normal temperature for a 4-year-old is 37.5–37.7° C (99.5°–99.9° F) so Sok Wu's temperature is below normal, probably the result of decreased tissue perfusion secondary to reduced oxygen intake. The normal pulse rate for a 3- to 5-year-old is 75–125 beats/minute. His pulse is elevated probably due to a combination of factors including anxiety, compensatory mechanism to increase cardiac output to compensate for decreasing tissue perfusion, and his mother and aunt's anxiety. His blood pressure is below the normal of 102/62. This also is the result of decreasing tissue perfusion caused by hypoxia. His oxygen

saturation is 78%, significantly below the normal range of 95% to 100%. The barely audible and diminished breath sounds indicate obstruction of the air entering and leaving the lungs, which would be expected in the presence of airway obstruction. The absence of crackles, rales, and rhonchi indicate that infection is probably not present. Stridor is a high-pitched sound made in the presence of air attempting to move through an obstruction of the trachea or larynx. The use of accessory muscles for breathing represents severe respiratory distress. The presence of weak and irregular heart sounds indicates that the heart is having difficulty compensating for decreased tissue perfusion. Cool and clammy skin may be a sign of impending shock as the body shunts blood from the extremities to redirect it to maintain perfusion of the vital organs of the heart and brain. His decreasing responsiveness probably is an indication of decreased tissue perfusion to the brain. All of these are consistently responses to foreign body aspiration resulting in decreased tissue perfusion.

4. **What are the nursing priorities for this situation?**
   a. Ineffective airway clearance related to the presence of a foreign body. The patency of the airway must be established and maintained.
   b. Risk for impaired gas exchange related to inability to inhale oxygen and exhale carbon dioxide secondary to foreign body aspiration
   c. Risk for ineffective tissue perfusion related to impaired gas exchange secondary to FBA
   d. Anxiety related to seriousness of child's condition and unfamiliar hospital surroundings
   e. Deficient knowledge related to child's condition, normal growth and development activities of preschooler, accident prevention

5. **Discuss how you think Sok Wu's mother and aunt are feeling at this point.** They are both very anxious and worried about Sok Wu and whether he can be successfully treated. They probably fear that he will die or suffer irreparable brain damage if he survives. They also are probably feeling guilty about leaving the uninflated balloons on the table where Sok Wu could pick one up. They are concerned about the other children at home. As an after thought, they may be concerned about letting the parents of the other children who were invited to the party know that the party has been canceled. This concern undoubtedly would be a fleeting one until Sok Wu's condition improves.

6. **The health care provider prescribes the following for Sok Wu:**

   Stat chest X-ray.
   Initiate PIV of 5% Dextrose and 0.2% normal saline to infuse at 70 mL/hour.
   Monitor oxygen saturation via pulse oximetry.

Maintain nothing by mouth (NPO).

Monitor continuous vital signs.

Following the chest X-ray which reveals a foreign body in his trachea, Sok Wu is scheduled for an emergency bronchoscopy. What is the rationale for this procedure in this case? Performing a bronchoscopy is a standard of care for a client with foreign body obstruction. It is performed to both positively identify the object and to remove it.

7. Following the successful bronchoscopy, what assessments should the nurse perform on Sok Wu? The nurse needs to monitor and maintain a patent airway; monitor vital signs hourly for at least 4 hours; monitor for return of the child's gag reflex which is anesthetized during the bronchoscopy; monitor the neurological status, breath sounds, heart sounds, skin temperature, and condition hourly; and monitor oxygen saturation via pulse oximetry continuously. As his condition improves, the assessments are performed less frequently and once the gag reflex returns, oral fluids are initiated and the nurse needs to assess the child's ability to swallow the fluids without choking. The nurse also needs to assess the child's level of growth and development and compare this with his normal. Assessments of the mother and aunt's interaction with Sok Wu should be performed.

8. The health care provider prescribes cefazolin 160 mg IV q6h × 3 doses with first dose to be administered stat. You asked the nursing assistant to weigh Sok Wu on the scales on his hospital bed as you communicate the medication order to pharmacy. The nursing assistant reports that Sok Wu weighs 16.5 kg (36.3 lb). Did the nurse act appropriately when she delegated obtaining Sok Wu's weight to the nursing assistant? Obtaining a client's weight is within the scope of practice for a nursing assistant and it was appropriate for the nurse to delegate this activity to the nursing assistant. The nurse needed to communicate the antibiotic prescription to pharmacy so it could be prepared and administered as soon as possible. This is a nursing responsibility and the nurse's focus at this point.

9. What process does the nurse use when administering medications to this child? The nursing process when administering medications to this or any client involves implementing the "7 rights."

RIGHT DRUG: Is this the drug that was prescribed and is this the right drug for this client?

Cefazolin is a first-generation cephalosporin that is prescribed following the removal of a foreign body to prophylactically prevent infection secondary to aspiration of an unsterile object. This drug's safety and efficacy have been proven for use in children. Administering three doses is typical prophylaxis.

RIGHT DOSE: Is this the dose that was prescribed and is this a safe dose for this client?

The safe dosage range for this drug when prescribed to a child is 25–100 mg/kg per day in four divided doses so each individual dose for Sok Wu is 103–412.5 mg. The dose prescribed for Sok Wu is safe for him based on his weight.

RIGHT CLIENT: Is this the right client for which this medication has been prescribed?

The nurse should check the health care provider's prescription and ensure it is on the client's medical record, compare the prescription to the medication administration record (MAR) of the child, compare the label on the minibag for the correct child's name, and check the name outside the child's hospital room. The final and most definitive identification is made by verifying the child's identification by his or her identification bracelet.

RIGHT TIME: Is this the correct time according to the prescription? Are the time intervals of administration appropriate for this drug and the route prescribed?

The first dose for Sok Wu was prescribed stat and should be administered as soon as possible. This drug is administered every 6 hours via the intravenous route.

RIGHT ROUTE: Is this the appropriate route to administer this medication? This drug is administered parenterally, usually by the intravenous route. The nurse also needs to validate that the vascular access is patent and free of complications. In addition, the rate of administration needs to be appropriate for the access. The time frame provided by the pharmacy for the rate of administration is the minimum time that it can be administered based on the drug's absorption, biotransformation, half-life, and elimination in and from the body. The nurse should base her rate of administration on the gauge of the intravenous catheter and the size of the vein where the access is located. Antimicrobials are very irritating to peripheral vessels and as a rule of thumb, should not be administered more than 25% greater than the rate of the maintenance intravenous fluids.

RIGHT DOCUMENTATION: The administration documentation should consist of the drug name, dose, route, and time of administration as well as the client's response. Medication administration should never be documented prior to administering the medication.

RIGHT TO REFUSE: The client has the right to refuse any medication; however, in the case of a child, this right usually rests with the parent or guardian of the child. Most refusals of medications are based on lack of or inaccurate information so the nurse needs to tell the client and significant other what the drug is and why it is being given prior to administration of each medication.

10. Describe your feelings about this situation considering Sok Wu's level of growth and development. Sok Wu is a preschooler who according to Erikson is involved in the developmental task of initiative versus guilt. His life revolves around socialization and imagination. Socialization provides the opportunity to initiate relationships beyond the immediate family unit. The associative play characteristic of this age group involves playing with other children of the same age. Initiative also can pose dangers to the child as his or her judgment concerning the safety of certain activities is not mature. Objects such as balloons fascinate the preschooler. Unfortunately, the child does not have the cognitive skills to understand the aspiration risk. The child's imagination provides for socialization when others are not present by the development of "imaginary friends." Unfortunately, the imagination can be the child's nemesis when the child is hospitalized and is responsible for his or her primary fear of mutilation at this time. This situation of FBA of balloons is a common threat for preschoolers in the presence of society's view that balloons are part of a child's birthday even in light of scientific evidence of the danger balloons pose to young children. The incidence of mortality from FBA in children is 350–2,000 annually with the peak incidence in children 1–3 years of age. The incidence is highest in boys under the age of 5 years. The most common aspirated objects are toys, of which balloons comprise 29% of deaths due to FBA. This is a preventable situation and parents of young children need to be educated about the dangers of balloons.

11. Thirty-six hours following his admission to the hospital, Sok Wu is discharged with no complications associated with his FBA. He is sent home with his mother and aunt. What would be the nurse's focus in discharge teaching for Sok Wu's mother and aunt?

    a. Assess the mother and aunt's knowledge of the situation.

    b. Reinforce information concerning growth and development and accident prevention.

    c. Provide verbal and written information regarding:

        (1) Medication administration, if appropriate

        (2) Signs and symptoms to report to health care provider

        (3) Contact numbers for questions

        (4) Importance of follow-up with health care provider

    d. Provide adequate time for mother and aunt to ask questions, answering them honestly.

    e. Document teaching and the mother and aunt's response.

References

Daniels, R. (2002). *Delmar's manual of laboratory and diagnostic tests.* Clifton Park, NY: Thomson Delmar Learning.

eMedicine article on *http://www.emedicine.com* by Munter, D.W. (2001). Foreign bodies, Trachea.

Gahart, B.L. and Nazareno, A.R. (2005). *2005 Intravenous medications* (21st ed.). St. Louis: Mosby.

North American Nursing Diagnosis Association. (2005). *Nursing diagnoses: Definitions & classifications, 2005–2006*. Philadelphia: NANDA.

Potts, N. and Mandleco, B. (2002). *Pediatric nursing: Caring for children and their families*. Clifton Park, NY: Thomson Delmar Learning.

Reiss, B.S., Evans, M.E., and Broyles, B. E. (2002). *Pharmacological aspects of nursing care*. (6th ed.). Clifton Park, NY: Thomson Delmar Learning, pp. 36–45.

Spratto, G.R. and Woods, A.L. (2005). *2005 Edition: PDR nurse's drug handbook*. Clifton Park, NY: Thomson Delmar Learning.

CASE STUDY 2

Steven

GENDER	**SOCIOECONOMIC**
M	■ Middle class
AGE	**SPIRITUAL**
7	
SETTING	**PHARMACOLOGIC**
■ School	■ Montelukast sodium (Singulair)
ETHNICITY	■ Beclomethasone (QUAR)
■ Native American	**PSYCHOSOCIAL**
CULTURAL CONSIDERATION	■ Routine exposure to second-hand smoke
	■ Anxiety
PREEXISTING CONDITIONS	**LEGAL**
■ Asthma	
COEXISTING CONDITION	**ETHICAL**
	■ Possible nurse bias
COMMUNICATION	**ALTERNATIVE THERAPY**
DISABILITY	**PRIORITIZATION**
	■ Yes
	DELEGATION

THE RESPIRATORY SYSTEM

Level of difficulty: Moderate

Overview: This case requires knowledge of reactive airway disease (RAD) asthma, the impact of second-hand smoke on respiratory ailments, growth and development, as well as an understanding of the client's background, personal situation, and parent–child relationship.

Client Profile

Steven Wolf is a 7-year-old boy who moved to Washington, DC 2 weeks ago with his parents and older brother Sean. His father is a government worker who has been transferred from his position in Colorado to a new government position in Washington, DC. Steven and his brother began the new school year this week, as did his mother who teaches third grade at another school in the same district. Steven was diagnosed with reactive airway disease (asthma) when he was 3 years old and is currently managed on montelukast 5 mg once a day and uses an beclomethasone inhaler approximately once a day for exacerbations. Both of his parents smoke 10–12 cigarettes a day at home.

Case Study

Steven experiences shortness of breath during recess at school and is brought to the school nurse's office after using his inhaler without relief. The school nurse notes that Steven's respirations are 30 breaths/minute; his heart rate is 125 beats/minute; he has audible wheezing; and his oxygen saturation via pulse oximetry is 90%. The nurse talks to Steven calmly, attempting to decrease his obvious anxiety while she continuously assesses his breathing, color, and level of consciousness. She has him sit in a high-back chair next to her desk, quickly reviews his medical history obtained when he registered to attend school, and then notifies his mother.

Questions

1. Discuss your impressions about the above situation using the data obtained.

2. Discuss the pathophysiology of reactive airway disease.

3. What pertinent information is missing?

4. What factors place Steven at risk for experiencing an "asthma attack"?

5. What is the relationship between Steven's condition and his oxygen saturation level?

6. Discuss why Steven is prescribed montelukast and beclomethasone for his asthma.

7. What is the normal dosage range of montelukast for Steven?

8. While assessing Steven, the school nurse asks him when he last used his beclomethasone inhaler. Why is this important information for the nurse as she attempts to assist Steven?

9. Discuss your feelings concerning parents who place their children at risk for health problems related to second-hand smoke.

10. Steven recovers from this episode of reactive airway. Discuss ways you might approach the client's parents about their cigarette smoking and the dangers it poses to Steven.

Questions and Suggested Answers

1. Discuss your impressions about the above situation using the data obtained. Steven's breathing pattern and history would suggest he is experiencing an "asthma attack" (an episode of hypoventilation). His vital signs are elevated from the normal values of a 7-year-old which should be pulse rate, 75–115 beats/minute and a respiratory rate of 18–24 breaths/minute. Wheezing is a cardinal manifestation of reactive airway disease due to bronchospasms as well as his oxygen saturation indicating hypoventilation.

2. Discuss the pathophysiology of reactive airway disease. Asthma is a hypersensitivity response in the airways causing them to be hyper reactive in response to exposure to irritants (usually airborne) that normally would not elicit a response. The smooth muscle of the bronchial tree in the person with asthma begins to spasm as a result of vagal nerve stimulation. This results in bronchoconstriction (see Fig. 2-1). In addition, the inflammatory response is stimulated as a result of the immunoglobulin E receptors triggering the mast cells to release histamine. This leads to edema that further narrows the airway. When the bronchi become inflamed, hypertrophied mucous glands secrete large amounts of thick mucus, which further impairs gas exchange. Additional biochemical mediators, such as leukotriene, interleukin-4, and exotoxin continue the inflammatory response and increase its duration. In addition to decreased oxygen passing through the airways to the lungs, carbon dioxide is trapped in the alveoli due to the airways normally being larger during inhalation than exhalation. Both of these lead to hyperventilation. Although this breathing pattern facilitates the release of carbon dioxide, the state of hypoxia resulting from decreased oxygen intake progresses to respiratory alkalosis. This leads to hypoventilation, recurrent respiratory acidosis, and eventual respiratory failure if the cycle persists.

3. What pertinent information is missing? Breath sounds, heart sounds, how often he uses his inhaler now, color of nailbeds and color around his lips, and following his transfer to a medical facility, arterial blood gases to measure acid–base balance.

4. What factors place Steven at risk for experiencing an "asthma attack"?
a. Moving to Washington, DC:

According to the United Press International's article of May 4, 2004, "The U.S. capital city has the highest rate of asthma in the nation, says the American Lung Association of Washington." It estimates that "10,000 children in Washington suffer from the disease." The article further states, "In addition to a poor ozone score (F), the region had poor grades for both short and year-round particle pollution, ranking it the 25th worst county in the nation for short-term particle pollution levels."

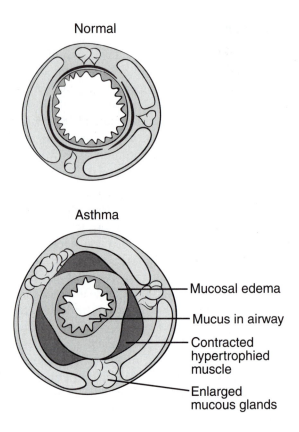

Figure 2-1 *Pathophysiology of asthma.*

b. Smoking habits of both of his parents:

Passive smoke has irritating airborne particles that research has shown decreases the anti-inflammation protein interleukin-10. This may contribute to the evidence showing a decreased level of interleukin-10 in children with asthma. Second-hand smoke is a known risk factor for the development of asthma in children.

c. Steven's age:

Asthma affects approximately 17 million persons in the United States. Children comprise 50% of this figure.

d. Stress:

Although stress is not a cause of asthma, it may serve as a catalyst for exacerbation. Steven has been uprooted from his home and former school at an age (school-age) when "best friends" and the need for accomplishment are highly influencing factors. His having to leave his friends and school in Colorado may increase his stress level. His current schoolmates may see him as different not only because he is new to the school, but also because he has trouble breathing and uses an inhaler. This may elicit unkind remarks from them, which would increase Steven's stress level.

5. What is the relationship between Steven's condition and his oxygen saturation level? This pathophysiologic response in asthma results in decreased oxygen intake, carbon dioxide retention, and hyperventilation as a compensatory mechanism. Prolonged hyperventilation leads to hypoventilation, resulting in the decrease of his oxygen saturation to 90% from the normal range of 95% to 100%.

6. Discuss why Steven is prescribed montelukast and beclomethasone inhaler for his asthma. Leukotrienes are responsible for increasing inflammation within the body, causing contraction of the airway muscle and increasing edema from the vasculature in the bronchi. Montelukast sodium is an antileukotriene and binds with the cysteinyl leukotriene receptors (associated with the symptoms of asthma) and prevents the action of cysteinyl leukotrienes. Beclomethasone is an inhaled corticosteroid that acts by decreasing the inflammation and edema that further decrease the lumen of the bronchi already narrowed by the bronchospasms.

7. What is the normal dosage range of montelukast for Steven? The standard dose of this agent for children aged 6 to 14 years is one 5-mg chewable tablet once daily at bedtime.

8. While assessing Steven, the school nurse asks him when he last used his beclomethasone inhaler. Why is this important information for the nurse as she attempts to assist Steven? Beclomethasone (Beconase) is a corticosteroid and in children 5–11 years of age, the recommended dose is 40 mcg twice a day. For Beconase the dose is one or two inhalations (42–84 mcg) in each nostril twice a day, not to exceed 160 mcg daily. This information helps the nurse assess how Steven has used his inhaler, if he understands his recommended dosing, or if he has taken too much or too little of the medication.

9. Discuss your feelings concerning parents who place their children at risk for health problems related to second-hand smoke. Nurses must be aware of their feelings and biases concerning lifestyles, especially those that impact health. This is necessary so the nurse can approach the parents therapeutically and not antagonize them by showing prejudices. If the parents are alienated, the chances that the nurse can positively impact on the situation will be dramatically diminished.

10. Steven recovers from this episode of reactive airway. Discuss ways you might approach the client's parents about their cigarette smoking and the dangers it poses to Steven. The nurse's approach must be both empathetic and therapeutic. She should understand that cigarette smoking and nicotine are addictions. Discussing the health hazards with Steven is important, as is providing literature concerning available smoking cessation programs. If the parents do not believe they can quit smoking at this time, encourage them to smoke outside the home and to avoid smoking in the car with Steven. It is essential that the nurse be nonjudgmental in her approach, including not expecting smokers to stop smoking abruptly after years of smoking. Providing them with support and information without judgment will encourage better compliance.

References

American Academy of Allergy Asthma and Immunology. *http://www.aaaai.org*

Broyles, B.E. (2005). *Medical-surgical clinical companion.* Durham, NC: Carolina Academic Press.

Centers for Disease Control. *http://www.cdc.gov*

Daniels, R. (2002). *Delmar's manual of laboratory and diagnostic tests.* Clifton Park, NY: Thomson Delmar Learning.

Gahart, B.L. and Nazareno, A.R. (2005). *2005 Intravenous medications* (21st ed.). St. Louis: Mosby.

Mayo Clinic. *http://www.mayoclinic.com*

MedlinePlus: Asthma. *http://www.nlm.nih.gov*

North American Nursing Diagnosis Association. (2005). *Nursing diagnoses: Definitions & classifications, 2005–2006.* Philadelphia: NANDA.

Potts, N. and Mandleco, B. (2002). *Pediatric nursing: Caring for children and their families.* Clifton Park, NY: Thomson Delmar Learning.

Spratto, G.R. and Woods, A.L. (2005). *2005 Edition: PDR Nurse's drug handbook.* Clifton Park, NY: Thomson Delmar Learning.

United Press International (2004) *Tuesday*, May 4, 2004: Washington has high asthma rate.

CASE STUDY 3

Kristin

GENDER	**SOCIOECONOMIC**
F	
AGE	**SPIRITUAL**
6 weeks old	
SETTING	**PHARMACOLOGIC**
■ Hospital	
ETHNICITY	**PSYCHOSOCIAL**
■ White American	■ Parental anxiety
CULTURAL CONSIDERATIONS	**LEGAL**
PREEXISTING CONDITIONS	**ETHICAL**
■ Preterm birth	
COEXISTING CONDITIONS	**ALTERNATIVE THERAPY**
COMMUNICATION	**PRIORITIZATION**
DISABILITY	**DELEGATION**
	■ Yes

DIFFICULT

THE RESPIRATORY SYSTEM

Level of difficulty: Difficult

Overview: This case requires knowledge of respiratory distress syndrome (RDS), growth and development, as well as an understanding of the client's background, personal situation, and parent–child attachment relationship.

Client Profile

Kristin is a 6-week-old infant who was born at 35 weeks' gestation and diagnosed with respiratory distress syndrome (RDS) shortly after birth. She is the third child in her family, which includes her 30-year-old parents, 4-year-old brother, and 2-year-old sister. Her mother developed gestational diabetes and in her 25th week of pregnancy developed preeclampsia. Although the treatment prescribed by her obstetrician was effective initially, her preeclampsia worsened during the 34th week and after a week of hospitalization, Kristin was delivered by caesarean section.

Case Study

On admission to the neonatal intensive care unit (NICU) immediately after birth, Kristin was manifesting a respiratory rate of 70 breaths/minute, expiratory grunting, nasal flaring, substernal retractions, and cyanosis in her hands and feet and around her mouth. Her admission arterial blood gases were: pH, 7.28; PCO_2, 50 mm Hg; PO_2, 40 mm Hg; oxygen saturation, 70%; and HCO_3, 20 mEq/L. She was placed on 100% oxygen, but when her respiratory rate and other manifestations did not improve within the first 30 minutes, surfactant replacement therapy was begun and she was placed on mechanical ventilation. She was removed from mechanical ventilation after 2 weeks and transferred to the intermediate care nursery last week. Her parents have visited every day since Kristin's birth but were unable to stay very long because of the two young children at home requiring childcare. Although both of Kristin's sets of grandparents have offered to stay with the children or have the children stay with them, her parents are reluctant to "impose" on them.

Questions

1. Discuss RDS, including the pathophysiology and other nomenclature for this condition.

2. Discuss the significance of Kristin's clinical manifestations.

3. Discuss the incidence of RDS and Kristin's risk factors for this condition.

4. Identify the potential complications associated with RDS.

5. What are the priorities of care for Kristin on admission to the neonatal intensive care unit after birth?

6. Discuss appropriate nursing interventions to meet the priorities of care for Kristin.

7. Discuss Kristin's treatment regimen including the rationales for these therapies.

8. Discuss your impressions of Kristin's parents' response to the offers of childcare.

9. Kristin's mother has been providing breast milk to the nursery for Kristin, who is now ingesting 30 mL of breast milk per bottle every 3 hours. The nurse discusses

with Kristin's mother that she can breastfeed Kristin as often as she likes. Kristin's
mother expresses concern that breastfeeding Kristin may tire the infant and cause
her to "have trouble breathing." Although
she is now able to stay with Kristin
throughout the day, she tells the nurse

that she can't stay 24 hours a day at the
hospital. How should the nurse respond
to the mother's concerns?

10. Kristin's parents and siblings are
preparing to take Kristin home. Discuss
the teaching priorities for them prior to
Kristin's discharge.

Questions and Suggested Answers

1. Discuss RDS including the pathophysiology and other nomenclature for this condition. RDS also is called infant respiratory distress syndrome (IRDS) and hyaline membrane disease. RDS is caused by a deficiency of surfactant, a complex lipoprotein needed to reduce the surface tension of the hyaline membranes that line the alveoli of the lungs and is most highly associated with preterm births. In the normal neonate, the hyaline membranes form within 30 minutes following birth, and within 2–3 days following birth surfactant is synthesized; however, in the preterm neonate, the hyaline membranes are immature and unable to produce adequate levels of surfactant. This lack of surfactant results in decreased lung compliance, residual capacity, and increased pulmonary dead space. As a result, the ventilation–perfusion ratio is mismatched and right-to-left shunting occurs. This can involve up to 80% of the neonate's cardiac output. Distal airways become distended and atelectasis occurs. As the pressure further distends the distal airways, the epithelial lining of the airways is injured, leading to the inflammatory process and exudates made of the fibrinous matrix from the blood. Hypoxia and respiratory acidosis result, which further interferes with surfactant synthesis.

2. Discuss the significance of Kristin's clinical manifestations. On admission to the neonatal intensive care unit (NICU), Kristin was exhibiting classic manifestations of RDS. She was tachypneic (normal respiratory rate in neonate is 35–50 breaths/minute) in an attempt to increase body oxygenation. Nasal flaring and sternal retractions are common in neonates experiencing respiratory distress because neonates are nose-breathers, so as they work harder to breathe, it is manifested by flaring of the nostrils and sternal retractions. Cyanosis represents hypoxia, as the tissues do not receive oxygen from the bloodstream and the tissues assume the cyanotic color. Expiratory grunting is another classic sign of respiratory distress and results from partial closure of the glottis. Her arterial blood gases indicate respiratory acidosis when compared to the normal values for a neonate: pH,

7.32–7.49; P_{CO_2}, 35–45 mm Hg; P_{O_2}, 60–70 mm Hg; oxygen saturation, 95% to 100%; and HCO_3, 20–26 mEq/L.

3. Discuss the incidence of RDS and Kristin's risk factors for this condition. Approximately 40,000 neonates in the United States are diagnosed with RDS annually. As many as 50% of neonates born between 28 and 32 weeks of gestation develop RDS. In those born before 28 weeks of gestation as many as 45% to 80% have RDS. It is more common in males. Risk factors: RDS occurs most commonly in preterm neonates. In addition, it is more common in infants born to women with diabetes and those delivered by caesarean section without experiencing labor (Pramanik, 2002).

4. Identify the potential complications associated with RDS. Potential complications of RDS include:
  a. Pulmonary
    (1) Atelectasis, pneumothorax
    (2) Pneumomediastinum
    (3) Bronchopulmonary dysplasia
  b. Cardiac
    (1) Patent ductus arteriosus
    (2) Hypotension
    (3) Decreased cardiac output
  c. Renal—decreased urinary output due to decreased renal perfusion
  d. Metabolic
    (1) Acidosis
    (2) Sodium imbalances
    (3) Hypocalcemia
    (4) Hypoglycemia
  e. Hematologic
    (1) Iron-deficiency anemia
    (2) DIC
  f. Neurological
    (1) Seizures
    (2) Increased intracranial pressure
    (3) Intraventricular hemorrhage
  g. Infection
  h. Retinopathy associated with increased supplemental oxygen levels

5. What are the priorities of care for Kristin on her admission to the neonatal intensive care unit after birth?
  a. Impaired gas exchange related to lack of surfactant and lung changes associated with RDS
  b. Ineffective airway clearance related to obstruction or displacement of the endotracheal tube

  c. Ineffective breathing pattern related to work of breathing to improve hypoxia

  d. Potential for injury related to complications of RDS and mechanical ventilation

  e. Risk for impaired parent–infant attachment related to Kristin's condition, required hospitalization, parental anxiety about leaving other siblings

  f. Deficient knowledge related to Kristin's condition, treatment, home care, and parental needs.

6. Discuss appropriate nursing interventions to meet her priorities of care.

  a. Gas exchange

   (1) Identify neonates at risk.

   (2) Monitor respiratory status via continuous cardiopulmonary monitoring.

   (3) Monitor oxygen saturation via pulse oximetry.

   (4) Monitor serial blood gases.

   (5) Position Kristin with head of bed elevated to support her ventilatory effort.

   (6) Monitor for manifestations of acid–base imbalances.

   (7) Administer oxygen as prescribed, titrating to prescribed oxygen saturation levels.

   (8) Initiate mechanical ventilation using prescribed parameters.

   (9) Administer sedation as prescribed to prevent Kristin from working against the ventilator.

   (10) Monitor ventilator setting and tubing at least hourly.

   (11) Provide chest physiotherapy as prescribed in collaboration with health care provider and respiratory therapy.

  b. Airway clearance

   (1) Assess breath sounds at least hourly and PRN as needed.

   (2) Reposition every 2 hours.

   (3) Provide in-line suctioning as needed.

  c. Breathing pattern

  Refer to Gas Exchange and Airway Clearance

  d. Risk for injury

   (1) Monitor serial arterial blood gases.

   (2) Check placement of endotracheal tube prior to placing Kristin on mechanical ventilation.

   (3) Reposition endotracheal tube per protocol to prevent damage to oral mucous membranes.

   (4) Provide mouth care every 2 hours and more frequently as needed.

      (5) Provide environment conducive to rest for Kristin.

      (6) Monitor for complications of RDS and mechanical ventilation.

  e. Parent–infant attachment

      (1) Encourage parental visitation with Kristin.

      (2) Encourage her parents to talk to her and gently stroke her.

      (3) Encourage parents to verbalize feelings and concerns.

      (4) As Kristin's condition allows, encourage parental participation in her care.

      (5) Have parents hold Kristin as soon as her condition allows.

      (6) Provide privacy (within the constraints of the critical care environment).

  f. Client teaching

      (1) Explain all procedures and equipment to Kristin's parents and repeat as needed.

      (2) Assess their knowledge of Kristin's condition.

      (3) Encourage them to ask questions and provide answers or referral for answers.

      (4) Discuss with Kristin's mother her preferences for infant feeding.

      (5) If her mother wants to breastfeed, provide information and equipment so she can pump.

      (6) Provide information concerning visitation to critical care unit and restrictions, as needed.

7. Discuss Kristin's treatment regimen including the rationales for these therapies. The first line of treatment for hypoxia is the administration of supplemental oxygen. According to Pramanik (2002), intrathecal surfactant replacement therapy is most effective when administered within 2 hours of birth. Mechanical ventilation is used to decrease the neonate's work of breathing and to provide adequate gas exchange. Mechanical ventilation also can help reverse atelectasis and pneumothorax. Nutritional support is begun following stabilization of the neonate's condition and may involve enteral feedings or total parenteral nutrition.

8. Discuss your impressions of Kristin's parents' response to the offers of childcare. Their response is normal, especially in this extremely stressful situation. They don't know how long Kristin will require hospitalization or even if she will survive. Because of normal feelings of powerlessness during this type of experience, returning home to their other children may provide them with a sense of normalcy and escape from the stressors of the hospital. We don't know the relationships between the parents and their parents; however, assuming it is functional, Kristin's parents simply may be concerned about imposing or if their parents are older or elderly, that the toddler and preschooler may be too much stress on them.

9. Kristin's mother has been providing breast milk to the nursery for Kristin who is now ingesting 30 mL of breast milk per bottle every 3 hours. The nurse discusses with Kristin's mother that she can breastfeed Kristin as often as she likes. Kristin's mother expresses concern that breastfeeding Kristin may tire the infant and cause her to "have trouble breathing." Although she is now able to stay with Kristin throughout the day, she tells the nurse that she can't stay 24 hours a day at the hospital. How should the nurse respond to the mother's concerns? Given Kristin's history, it is normal for her mother to be concerned about tiring her out by breastfeeding her. She should be told that Kristin's health care provider has prescribed that she can breastfeed and that the nurse will be monitoring Kristin during the feedings. She also should be told that if Kristen is unable to complete her feeding at the breast, the remainder of the feeding can be provided by bottle. Kristin's mother's concerns about not being able to stay for 24 hours is understandable; however the nurse should explain that, if she wishes, she can breastfeed during the day and the nursing staff will feed Kristin the pumped and bottled breast milk when her mother is unable to be there. These are both common practices in the neonatal and intermediate care nurseries.

10. Kristin's parents and siblings are preparing to take Kristin home. Discuss the teaching priorities for them prior to Kristin's discharge.
   a. Assess her parents' level of understanding about Kristin's present condition
   b. Provide verbal and written information (and demonstrations and return demonstrations as needed) concerning:
      (1) Infant care including bathing, feeding, positioning
      (2) Signs and symptoms of respiratory distress
      (3) Contact numbers to report signs and symptoms or for questions they may have
      (4) How to use respiratory monitor if prescribed for home use
      (5) Infant cardiopulmonary resuscitation
      (6) Developmental milestones and that Kristin will require time to compensate for her prematurity
      (7) Importance of follow-up management
   c. Provide adequate time for questions, return demonstrations as needed.
   d. Document teaching and parental response, noting that discharge teaching should begin on admission.

References

Centers for Disease Control. *http://www.cdc.gov*
Daniels, R. (2002). *Delmar's manual of laboratory and diagnostic tests.* Clifton Park, NY: Thomson Delmar Learning, p. 109.

McKinney, E.S., James, S.R., Murray, S.S., and Ashwill, J.W. (2005). Maternal-child nursing (2nd ed.).St. Louis: Elsevier Sunders, p. 648.

National Lung, Heart, and Blood Institute of the National Institutes of Health. *http://www.nlhb.nih.gov*

North American Nursing Diagnosis Association. (2005). *Nursing diagnoses: Definitions & classifications, 2005–2006.* Philadelphia: NANDA.

Potts, N. and Mandleco, B. (2002). *Pediatric nursing: Caring for children and their families.* Clifton Park, NY: Thomson Delmar Learning, p. 732.

Pramanik, A. (2002). Respiratory distress syndrome. *http://www.emedicine.com*

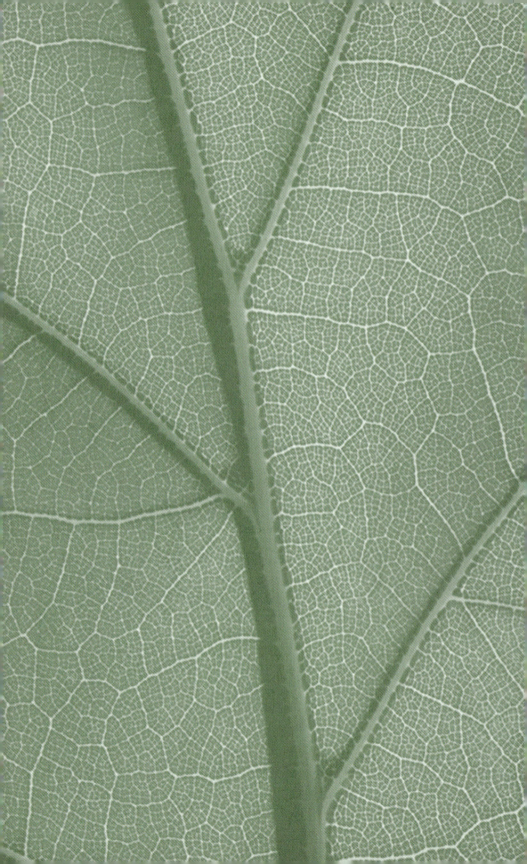

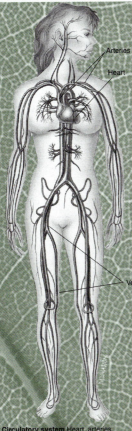

PART THREE

Arteries

Heart

Veins

Circulatory system Heart, arteries, veins, capillaries and blood.

The Cardiovascular System and the Blood

Candy

GENDER

F

AGE

13

SETTING

- Home/health care provider's office

ETHNICITY

- White American

CULTURAL CONSIDERATIONS

PREEXISTING CONDITIONS

- Menstruation

COEXISTING CONDITIONS

COMMUNICATION

DISABILITY

SOCIOECONOMIC

SPIRITUAL

PHARMACOLOGIC

- Ferrous sulfate (Feosol)

PSYCHOSOCIAL

- Single parent
- Anxiety

LEGAL

ETHICAL

ALTERNATIVE THERAPY

PRIORITIZATION

DELEGATION

- Client teaching

THE CARDIOVASCULAR SYSTEM

Level of difficulty: Easy

Overview: This case requires knowledge of iron-deficiency anemia (IDA), nutrition, growth and development, as well as an understanding of the client's background, personal situation, and family relationship.

Client Profile

Candy is a 13-year-old who lives with her father and younger sister. Her mother died when Candy was 6 years old and her sister was 4 years old. Her father works a 12-hour shift full-time to support himself and his daughters, and Candy makes sure she and her sister get to school each morning, take care of the house after school, and prepare their father's dinner so he can eat as soon as he gets home from work. All three are very close and on his days off, Candy's father is very devoted to his children. Candy began her menses when she was 11 years old and experiences regular periods every 28 days. She has excelled in school, being on the honor rolls consistently for the past 3 years. The past semester Candy's school performance began to decline and she has been complaining of being tired "all of the time." Her father notes that Candy "looks pale" and makes an appointment for Candy to see her pediatrician.

Case Study

At the pediatrician's office, the nurse performs a nursing history during which Candy's father shares the observations he has made and Candy verifies the information. The nurse's assessment reveals Candy is a clean, appropriately dressed, pale adolescent who appears fatigued. Candy's vital signs are:

Temperature: 35.9° C (96.6° F)
Pulse: 116 beats/minute
Respirations: 30 breaths/minute
Blood pressure: 90/60
Candy's lab values are:
Hemoglobin: 10 g/dL
Hematocrit: 28%
TIBC: 450 mg/dL
Serum iron: 35 µg/L

Questions

1. What are your impressions of this situation?

2. Discuss the pathophysiology and risk factors for iron-deficiency anemia (IDA).

3. Is there a relationship between Candy's change in school performance and her diagnosis?

4. Discuss the relationship between Candy's clinical manifestations and IDA.

5. Discuss the significance of Candy's laboratory values.

6. Discuss the cause-and-effect relationship between Candy's level of growth and development and her diagnosis.

7. What other assessment data would be helpful for the nurse to have to prepare Candy's teaching plan?

8. What are the priorities of care for Candy?

9. Candy is prescribed ferrous sulfate 300 mg t.i.d. What are the teaching priorities for Candy and her mother related to this prescription? What is the significance of the teaching plan?

10. What other responsibilities of care are delegated to Candy and her father in the teaching plan?

11. How can the nurse evaluate the effectiveness of the teaching done with Candy and her father?

Questions and Suggested Answers

1. What are your impressions of this situation? Candy and her family seem to have a very loving relationship; however, Candy and her sister are left on their own on the days their father works. Their father, Mr. Engle, spends time with them when he isn't working and seems devoted to them. From the profile and clinical manifestations, Candy appears to have iron-deficiency anemia (IDA).

2. Discuss the pathophysiology and risk factors for IDA. Iron is a mineral necessary for the synthesis of hemoglobin. Hemoglobin, a crystallizable, conjugated protein, is responsible for carrying oxygen from the lungs to the body tissues. In the lungs it combines with oxygen to form oxyhemoglobin. In the tissues, the oxyhemoglobin exchanges its oxygen for carbon dioxide. The most common source of iron is the diet and recycled old red blood cells. Although the bone marrow continues to manufacture erythrocytes on which the hemoglobin travels, their function is inadequate because of the insufficient amount of iron available. This process leads to the clinical manifestations of inadequate tissue perfusion. IDA develops gradually after the normal body stores of iron have been depleted.

Risk factors for developing IDA include inadequate intake of iron-rich foods and vitamin C (increases the absorption of iron), blood loss from natural (menses) or disease conditions (gastrointestinal bleeding disorders, malabsorption disorders). IDA affects 20% of American women and is much more common in cultures that lack adequate nutrition.

3. Is there a relationship between Candy's change in school performance and her diagnosis? The central nervous system is the most sensitive in the body to decreases in blood oxygen. IDA causes cognitive functioning to decrease as a result of insufficient oxygen for neuron function. Candy's change in school performance is evidence of this process.

4. Discuss the relationship between Candy's clinical manifestations and IDA. As a result of decreased hemoglobin, fatigue occurs because the cells and tissues in the body do not have adequate oxygen to meet their metabolic needs. Fatigue results as well as a decrease in body temperature because of the slowing of metabolism. In response to cellular demand for oxygen, the heart works harder, as evidenced by Candy's tachycardia, to increase cardiac output. The lungs work harder, as evidenced by Candy's tachypnea, in conjunction with the heart. Hemoglobin also helps maintain blood pressure by adding oxyhemoglobin to the red blood cells. Hypotension occurs with the decrease in vascular volume. Normal vital signs for Candy are temperature, 36.6° C (97.9° F); pulse, 60–110 beats/minute; respirations, 14–20 breaths/minute; and blood pressure, 118–121/76–80. Further, hemoglobin gives the red blood cells their deep red color which is responsible for the normal color of the Caucasian skin.

5. Discuss the significance of Candy's laboratory values. Normal blood values for Candy are the same as those for adult females and include:

Hemoglobin: 12–16 g/dL
Hematocrit: 38% to 47%
Total iron binding capacity: 300–360 mg/dL
Serum iron: 65–165 µg/L

Candy's lab values indicate anemia and her TIBC and serum iron values represent that inadequate iron is the cause of the anemia.

6. Discuss the cause-and-effect relationship between Candy's level of growth and development and her diagnosis. Although fatigue is not uncommon in adolescence because of the growth spurt occurring during these years, anemia is not a normal disorder for this age group. In addition, Candy is experiencing blood loss monthly through menstruation that can lead to IDA if her diet does not include adequate sources of iron and vitamin C. Dietary changes are common in adolescence as a result of increased metabolic demands, peer pressure, increased social activity, fad diets including decreasing intake of red meat (the best source of dietary iron), as well as, for adolescent girls, the pressure to be thin. Her fatigue probably also interferes with the amount of energy she has to eat. In addition, her fatigue and decreased school performance probably negatively impact on her activities with peers. Because peers provide adolescents with their primary source of belonging, IDA can have undesired effects on Candy's struggle for independence. Her responsibilities at home also may impact on her time with friends.

7. What other assessment data would be helpful for the nurse to have to prepare Candy's teaching plan?
   a. Nutrition history
   b. Platelet count
   c. White blood cell count
   d. Detailed menstruation history

8. **What are the priorities of care for Candy?**
   a. Ineffective tissue perfusion related to decreased oxygen-carrying capacity of the blood
   b. Imbalanced nutrition: less than body requirements related to inadequate intake of iron-rich foods
   c. Deficient knowledge related to nutritional needs for Candy, her condition, and treatment

9. **Candy is prescribed ferrous sulfate 300 mg t.i.d. What are the teaching priorities for Candy and her father related to this prescription? What is the significance of the teaching plan?** They need to know that ferrous sulfate is an oral iron supplement that will help treat Candy's condition. The nurse must review the prescription to be sure Candy and her father know the correct dose and how often the medication must be taken each day. Candy must receive adequate vitamin C in her diet to increase the absorption of the iron. Finally, the nurse needs to discuss the common adverse effects of this medication, including gastrointestinal upset, diarrhea, constipation, abdominal cramping and nausea, and black stools as well as interventions to reduce these effects. Taking iron with meals helps decrease the gastric distress and adequate intake of 2,500–3,000 mL of fluid each will help prevent constipation. If diarrhea occurs, the health care provider should be notified.

10. **What other responsibilities of care are delegated to Candy and her father in the teaching plan?**
    a. Following assessment of Candy's food preferences, nutrition instructions about iron-rich foods, amount of helpings needed per week
    b. Understanding of the risk factors for Candy and how to prevent these from into developing IDA
    c. Signs and symptoms to report to her health care provider
    d. Importance of follow-up with the health care provider

11. **How can the nurse evaluate the effectiveness of the teaching done with Candy and her father?** Assessing Candy's eye contact and interest level during the teaching sessions will help the nurse determine Candy's readiness for teaching, which greatly impacts the amount and accuracy of the material Candy hears. Candy and her father should be asked to repeat the instructions back to the nurse including how Candy will adjust her routine to be compliant with the treatment regimen. Follow-up phone communications with Candy by the nurse can help the nurse evaluate the effectiveness of the teaching. Finally, keeping follow-up appointments and the follow-up laboratory values are the most objective measures of Candy's compliance.

References

Centers for Disease Control. *http://www.cdc.gov*

Daniels, R. (2002). *Delmar's manual of laboratory and diagnostic tests.* Clifton Park, NY: Thomson Delmar Learning.

National Heart, Lung, and Blood Institute. *http://www.nhlb.nih.gov*

North American Nursing Diagnosis Association. (2005). *Nursing diagnoses: Definitions & classifications, 2005–2006.* Philadelphia: NANDA.

Potts, N. and Mandleco, B. (2002). *Pediatric nursing: Caring for children and their families.* Clifton Park, NY: Thomson Delmar Learning, pp. 812–818.

Spratto, G.R. and Woods, A.L. (2005). *2005 Edition: PDR nurse's drug handbook.* Clifton Park, NY: Thomson Delmar Learning, pp. 663–666.

C A S E   S T U D Y   2

Adriana

GENDER	**SOCIOECONOMIC**
F	
AGE	**SPIRITUAL**
7	
SETTING	**PHARMACOLOGIC**
■ Clinic	■ Deferoxamine mesylate (Desferal)
ETHNICITY	**PSYCHOSOCIAL**
■ Mediterranean	■ Effects of frequent and continued hospitalizations
CULTURAL CONSIDERATIONS	**LEGAL**
PREEXISTING CONDITIONS	**ETHICAL**
■ Beta-Thalassemia	
COEXISTING CONDITIONS	**ALTERNATIVE THERAPY**
■ Hemosiderosis	
COMMUNICATION	**PRIORITIZATION**
DISABILITY	**DELEGATION**

MODERATE

THE BLOOD

Level of difficulty: Moderate

Overview: This case requires knowledge of beta-thalassemia, treatment and complications, growth and development, as well as an understanding of the client's background, personal situation (living with chronic condition), and parent–child relationship.

Client Profile

Adriana is a 7-year-old who lives with her parents in a suburban community. Her parents brought Adriana to the United States from their homeland in Greece when she was 1 year old. At the age of 3, Adriana was in the 10th percentile for height and weight, pale, and her hemoglobin was 5.8 g/dL. Following further diagnostic studies, she was diagnosed with beta-thalassemia major. Over the course of the next 4 years, Adriana was hospitalized every 1–2 months so she could be transfused with packed red blood cells.

Case Study

During a routine follow-up visit at the hematology clinic, Adriana's laboratory results were as follows:

Hemoglobin: 10 mg/dL
Total serum iron: 150 µg/L

The hematologist discusses the planned treatment with Adriana and her parents.

Questions

1. Discuss the significance of Adriana's family's geographical background to her diagnosis.

2. What is beta-thalassemia, its incidence and etiology?

3. Discuss the clinical manifestations of beta-thalassemia.

4. Discuss the significance of Adriana's laboratory values.

5. Discuss the complications associated with the chronic blood transfusions associated with Adriana's condition.

6. Discuss the standards of care once Adriana reaches the parameters prescribed for annual packed red blood

cell transfusions and how it affects the child's need for future blood transfusions.

7. What are the priorities of care for Adriana?

8. Adriana is diagnosed with hemosiderosis. What is hemosiderosis and how is it treated?

9. Adriana is prescribed an initial dose of deferoxamine mesylate 1 g IM and 400 mg SC each day for 5 days. Adriana weighs 15 kg (33 lb). Would the nurse question this prescription?

10. Discuss the options available for Adriana to prevent lifelong blood transfusions.

Questions and Suggested Answers

1. Discuss the significance of Adriana's family's geographical background to her diagnosis. Beta-thalassemia is an autosomal recessive genetic disorder affecting hemoglobin chains and has its highest incidence in children

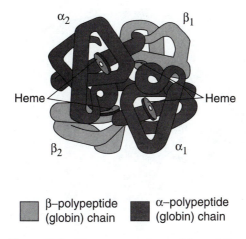

α_2 β_1

Heme ◄──────────► Heme

β_2 α_1

█ β–polypeptide   █ α–polypeptide
  (globin) chain   (globin) chain

Figure 3-1   *The structure of normal hemoglobin.*

of Mediterranean descent. The primary populations are Italian, Greek, and Syrian. With the increased influx of immigrants into the United States, the incidence of thalassemia is increasing.

2.   What is beta-thalassemia, its incidence and etiology? Normally the hemoglobin is made up of globin chains (Hb-α and Hb-β) (see Fig. 3-1). In beta-thalassemia the beta chains of the molecule of the hemoglobin are missing. This results in deficient hemoglobin and the development of fragile, microcytic, hypochromic erythrocytes. These erythrocytes are unable to carry adequate oxygen to the cells and tissue, leading to inadequate tissue perfusion and delayed growth and development. According to the Cooley's Anemia Foundation, there are three types of beta-thalassemia and their effects on the body range from mild to severe. Thalassemia minor, also referred to as thalassemia trait, lacks the beta protein but not sufficiently to interfere with the normal functioning of the body's hemoglobin. A person with thalassemia minor simply has the genetic trait. Thalassemia intermedia is a "condition (where) the lack of beta protein in the hemoglobin is great enough to cause a moderately severe anemia and significant health problems, including bone deformities and enlargement of the spleen." The severity of this condition is measured by the number of blood transfusions the child requires. "Generally speaking, patients with thalassemia intermedia need blood transfusions to improve their quality of life, but not in order to survive." Finally, beta-thalassemia major is the most severe form of this disease "in which the complete lack of beta protein in the hemoglobin causes a life-threatening anemia that requires regular blood transfusions and extensive ongoing medical care." Enlargement of both the spleen and liver and jaundice resulting from increased hemolysis of the abnormal red blood cells is common. The stress placed on the bone marrow to increase production of erythrocytes for tissue

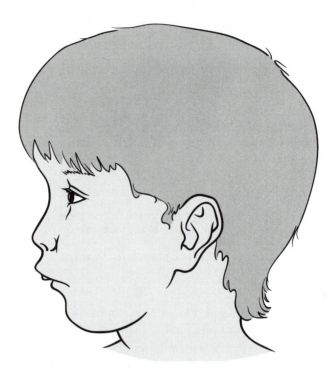

Figure 3-2   *Face of a child with beta-Thalessemia. Note the unusual features, including prominent and protruding forehead and flattened nose, caused by expansion of the facial bones to accommodate hyperplastic marrow.*

perfusion causes hyperplasia of the bone marrow that leads to thickening of the bones throughout the body and delayed development.

Thalassemias are most dominant in certain Eastern European populations. Individuals of Mediterranean descent are more likely to have deficient beta-globulin thalassemia. This condition also is referred to as Cooley's anemia or Mediterranean anemia. Both Africans and African-Americans also have an increased incidence of thalassemia.

The incidence of thalassemia varies worldwide; however, more than 1,500 people in the United States are affected and 2 million carry the genetic traits for thalassemia. Thalassemia is an autosomal recessive genetic disorder, and those with the disease have a usual life span of 20–30 years.

3. Discuss the clinical manifestations of beta-thalassemia. The clinical manifestations are the direct result of the pathophysiologic process of thalassemia. Pallor is present because hemoglobin is a major factor in the normal skin color. Children with thalassemia are usually small for their age, reaching only the 5th percentile for growth. They experience recurrent severe anemia (hemoglobin < 6 g/dL) and hepatosplenomegaly. The stress on the bone marrow causes the bones to thicken and become less flexible (see Fig. 3-2). This leads to pathological fractures and pain.

4. Discuss the significance of Adriana's laboratory values. Adriana is experiencing anemia as indicated by her hemoglobin level of 10 g/dL; however, for children with beta-thalassemia, the goal of treatment is to maintain hemoglobin levels between 9 and 10 g/dL. The more disturbing value is her total serum iron of 150 μg/L. The normal level of serum iron for children is 50–120 μg/L. Adriana's value indicates iron toxicity.

5. Discuss the complications associated with the chronic blood transfusions in Adriana's condition. The primary complication of chronic blood transfusions is elevated iron levels that can lead to tissue and organ failure.

6. Discuss the standards of care once Adriana reaches the parameters prescribed for annual packed red blood cell transfusions and how they affect the child's need for future blood transfusions. The standard of care once Adriana reaches the parameters for annual red blood cell transfusions is the removal of the spleen. The spleen enlarges, resulting in increased hemolysis of red blood cells. This process increases the risk and progression of iron toxicity. A splenectomy results in a lifelong increased risk for infection, requiring the use of prophylactic antibiotics.

7. What are the priorities of care for Adriana?
   a. Inaeffective tissue perfusion related to deficiency of hemoglobin secondary to disease process
   b. Risk for injury, tissue and organ damage related to elevated serum iron levels
   c. Deficient knowledge related to Adriana's condition, treatment, and home care

8. Adriana is diagnosed with hemosiderosis. What is hemosiderosis and how is it treated? Hemosiderosis is the term for elevated serum iron levels. It occurs as a result of chronic blood transfusions and is treated with the use of a chelating agent. Deferoxamine mesylate is the agent of choice to reduce serum iron levels.

9. Adriana is prescribed an initial dose of deferoxamine mesylate 1 g IM and 400 milligrams SC each day for 5 days. Adriana weighs 33 lb. Would the nurse question this prescription? As noted above, deferoxamine mesylate is the chelating agent of choice to treat iron toxicity caused by chronic blood transfusions. The normal loading dose of this agent is 1 g either intramuscularly or intravenously. It is then prescribed based on 20–40 mg/kg per day administered by subcutaneous mini-infusion pump over a period of 8–24 hours. The usual duration of treatment is 5–7 days. Adriana can receive 300–600 mg of this agent per day so her dose is safe and although the nurse would evaluate the prescription based on the 7 rights of medication administration, she would not question this prescription.

10. Discuss the options available for Adriana to prevent the need for life-long blood transfusions. Either bone marrow transplantation (BMT) or cord blood transplantation is indicated to prevent the lifelong need for blood transfusions. BMTs are complicated by the need for the donor to be genetically matched to the recipient. Cord blood transplants are similar to BMTs except the stem cells are harvested from the placenta or umbilical cord of a suitable donor. The advantage of cord blood transplants is that the donor does not require as close a genetic match as for BMT and the probability of rejection is much lower.

References

Cooley's Anemia Foundation. *http://www.thalassemia.org*

Centers for Disease Control. *http://www.cdc.gov*

Daniels, R. (2002). *Delmar's manual of laboratory and diagnostic tests.* Clifton Park, NY: Thomson Delmar Learning.

Gahart, B.L. and Nazareno, A.R. (2005). *2005 Intravenous medications* (21st ed.). St. Louis: Mosby.

North American Nursing Diagnosis Association. (2005). *Nursing diagnoses: Definitions & classifications, 2005–2006.* Philadelphia: NANDA.

Potts, N. and Mandleco, B. (2002). *Pediatric nursing: Caring for children and their families.* Clifton Park, NY: Thomson Delmar Learning, pp. 824–826.

Spratto, G.R. and Woods, A.L. (2005). *2005 Edition: PDR nurses' drug handbook.* Clifton Park, NY: Thomson Delmar Learning, pp. 507–508.

Wong, D.L., Perry, S.E., and Hockenberry, M.J. (2002). *Maternal child nursing care* (2nd ed.). St. Louis: Mosby, pp. 1364–1365.

CASE STUDY 3

Kevin

GENDER	**SOCIOECONOMIC**
M	
AGE	**SPIRITUAL**
8	
SETTING	**PHARMACOLOGIC**
■ Hospital	■ Lactated Ringer's solution
ETHNICITY	**PSYCHOSOCIAL**
■ White American	■ Anxiety
CULTURAL CONSIDERATIONS	**LEGAL**
PREEXISTING CONDITIONS	**ETHICAL**
COEXISTING CONDITIONS	**ALTERNATIVE THERAPY**
COMMUNICATION	**PRIORITIZATION**
■ Client is nonresponsive	
DISABILITY	**DELEGATION**
	■ Referrals

THE CARDIOPULMONARY SYSTEM

Level of difficulty: Difficult

Overview: This case requires knowledge of shock, growth and development, as well as an understanding of the client's background, personal situation, and family–child relationship.

Client Profile

Kevin is an 8-year-old school-age child who lives with his parents and two older brothers, ages 14 and 16. Kevin's brothers take care of him after school until his parents come home about 5:30 P.M. Kevin plays outdoors with his friends after school each day in his back yard. His brothers are very responsible and keep close watch over their younger brother. Today is the awards presentations at school immediately following classes and his mother and brothers attend the ceremony. Because their mother is driving Kevin home, his brothers have the opportunity to spend time with their friends and their father will pick them up after work. As Kevin and his mother are driving home, a large truck runs a red light, hitting their vehicle in the side where Kevin is sitting and causing multiple trauma to Kevin. His mother receives some contusions and abrasions and is taken to the hospital by the EMS with Kevin. Both were wearing seat restraints.

Case Study

Kevin is admitted to the pediatric intensive care unit (PICU) in critical condition. After his brief admission assessment, he has an intravenous infusion of lactated Ringer's solution at 200 mL/hour. His admitting diagnosis is multiple trauma and shock. He is placed on cardiopulmonary monitoring, mechanical ventilation, pulse oximetry monitoring, has a central venous access and an arterial line established, and a nasogastric tube and indwelling urinary catheter placed. His vital signs on admission were:

Temperature: 35° C (95° F)
Pulse: 130 beats/minute
Respirations: 45 breaths/minute and labored
Blood pressure: 110/50.

Questions

1. Discuss the significance of Kevin's vital signs.

2. Discuss the pathophysiology of shock.

3. Discuss the types and stages of shock and what type and stage you think Kevin is experiencing.

4. What complications can occur as a result of shock?

5. What other assessment data would be helpful for the nurse to have to prepare Kevin's care plan?

6. What are the priorities of care for Kevin on admission?

7. Discuss the rationales for Kevin's intravenous fluid prescription.

8. What is the rationale for placing Kevin on mechanical ventilation?

9. Discuss the purpose of the placement of Kevin's central venous access and arterial line.

10. Discuss the rationale for both continuous pulse oximetry and arterial blood gas monitoring.

11. What is the health care provider's rationale for placing a nasogastric tube and an indwelling urinary catheter?

12. Kevin's parents stay at his bedside constantly. His mother says to you, "I am so afraid my baby is not going to make it and it's all my fault. If I had just been watching the traffic closer, maybe this never would have happened." She weeps as her husband tries to console her. How can you therapeutically respond to Kevin's mother?

13. Kevin's brothers visit him regularly and even though he is not responsive, they talk to him about school and bring him cards and messages from his classmates. They bring in a CD player and play some of the current music. Discuss the potential effects of his brothers' visits.

14. Kevin's mother actively participates in his activities of daily living (ADLs) including bathing, mouth care, and range-of-motion. Discuss the importance of Kevin's mother participating in Kevin's care.

15. After 1 week in pediatric intensive care, Kevin's mean arterial pressure is 90 mm Hg and his is being weaned from mechanical ventilation. His oxygen saturation is 100% on 30% oxygen. Discuss the significance of these findings.

16. Kevin's condition has stabilized and is being prepared for transfer to the pediatric surgical unit. He complains of being tired and according to his parents, "He has been so cranky lately even though he's been getting better." Discuss your impression of Kevin's behavior.

17. On the nursing unit, referrals are made to the hospital school and recreation therapy for Kevin. Discuss the rationale for these referrals.

Questions and Suggested Answers

1. **Discuss the significance of Kevin's vital signs.** The most common cause of shock in children is multiple trauma. Kevin's vital signs indicate that he is in the compensatory stage of shock during which the heart rate and respiratory rate increase in response to the "fight-or-flight" mechanism that the body undergoes following trauma. His temperature is below normal and his skin is cool and clammy, representing the shunting of blood from the periphery to the vital organs of the heart and brain. His blood pressure is within normal limits, indicating that he has lost <40% of his circulating blood volume and that, at least for now, the compensatory mechanisms designed to maintain blood pressure are successful.

2. **Discuss the pathophysiology of shock.** The cardiovascular system is comprised of three major components: (1) blood volume, (2) cardiac pump, and (3) vasculature. Shock is hypoperfusion and occurs when one or more of these components malfunction, causing cellular effects that are triggered by the decreased blood supply to the cells. The reduction in oxygen results in decreased cellular ability to metabolize energy and depletes levels of adenosine triphosphate (ATP). ATP is stored energy necessary for the performance of cellular functions, such as biochemical synthesis for electrical conduction, muscular contraction, and active transport. ATP can

be synthesized both aerobically and anaerobically; however, aerobic metabolism is more efficient, yielding increased amounts of ATP per mole of glucose. Because of the decreased circulating oxygen supply to the cells in shock, aerobic metabolism decreases and anaerobic increases. Anaerobic metabolism not only is less efficient in producing energy but also produces lactic acid as a toxic byproduct of this type of metabolism. Increased lactic acid levels create an acidic cellular environment, causing decreased cellular function, cellular swelling, increased cellular permeability, and metabolic acidosis. The increased cellular permeability leads to impairment of the sodium–potassium pump as electrolytes flow freely in and out of the cells, causing structural damage to the cells and eventually cell death. Initially in the shock response, the body attempts to compensate for this hypoperfusion by stimulation of the sympathetic nervous system causing a release of catecholamines. This results in vasoconstriction, increasing the cardiopulmonary rates and cardiac contractility to increase cardiac output and maintain mean arterial pressure and blood pressure. In addition, blood is shunted from other areas of the body to the heart, lungs, and brain to maintain vital functions. Vascular responses include activation of central regulatory mechanisms that cause dilation and constriction to maintain the blood pressure. Local regulatory mechanisms cause vasoconstriction and vasodilation in response to chemicals released by the cells that communicate their need for oxygen and nutrients. Metabolic acidosis occurs as a result of cellular anaerobic metabolism stimulating the pulmonary acid–base buffer system, resulting in an increased respiratory rate in an effort to blow off carbon dioxide (CO_2). This response raises blood pH, causing respiratory alkalosis leading to mental status changes (confusion and combativeness). Among the areas from which blood is shunted is the kidneys, to retain fluid by preventing fluid excretion. Blood also is shunted from the gastrointestinal tract to decrease metabolic needs of this high energy consuming system. Further, blood is shunted from the periphery. If the compensatory responses are ineffective and the shock response is not reversed, multiple organ failure including heart ischemia and cardiac dysrhythmias occurs and death results.

3.   Discuss the types and stages of shock and what type and stage you think Kevin is experiencing. Hypovolemic shock is the most common type of shock and is caused by a marked decrease in intravascular volume. Cardiogenic shock occurs when pathology causes the heart to become ineffective as a pump. Vasogenic or distributive shock occurs when massive vasodilatation in the vessels occurs, leading to a maldistribution of blood volume. Finally, obstructive shock results indirectly from cardiac pump failure secondary to a condition that obstructs blood supply to the heart. The shock response occurs over a continuum of phases: (1) initial, (2) compensatory phase, (3) progressive, and (4) irreversible. Most students want a specific time frame for shock; however, the time progression through the stages of shock is directly proportional to the severity of the underlying cause. Regardless of the type of shock, the initial stage occurs at the cellular level in response to hypoperfusion. Generally clinical manifestations do not occur during this stage. Following this initial response, the compensatory stage is stimulated and the focus of this stage is to increase cardiac output to maintain blood pressure and mean arterial pressure to the brain and heart. If hypoperfusion continues, the client moves into the progressive stage of shock because the mechanisms for maintaining blood pressure and mean arterial pressure (MAP) are ineffective. During this stage, the blood pressure begins to drop and all organs including the heart and brain experience hypoperfusion. The heart is overworked trying to compensate. This leads to heart ischemia and cardiac dysrhythmias, causing the heart to pump ineffectively. Relaxation of precapillary sphincters cause leakage of fluid from the capillaries that decreases vascular fluid return to the heart. Decreased cardiac output results. As the shunting of blood initiated in the compensatory stage progresses, renal, liver, and gastrointestinal function decreases and ischemia occurs. This places the client at a high risk for infection and decreasing ability to metabolize and excrete medications and waste products such as ammonia and lactic acid or to filter out bacteria. Gastrointestinal (GI) ischemia leads to stress ulcers in the stomach and increased risk of GI bleed. Hematologic instability including sluggish blood flow, hypotension, and metabolic acidosis can result in disseminated intravascular dissemination (DIC). Finally, if shock continues to progress, the client will experience the irreversible stage of shock that represents the point along the shock continuum when organ damage is so extensive that the organs do not respond to treatment and the client is unable to survive. Multiple trauma in children usually causes hypovolemic shock except in the case of a head injury where neurogenic shock will occur. His vital signs indicate that he is in the compensatory stage of shock as he has tachycardia; tachypnea; and cool, clammy skin (shunting of blood from the periphery), but his blood pressure is within normal limits for his age and growth and development. However, his oxygen saturation indicates hypoxia secondary to hypoperfusion.

4. **What complications can occur as a result of shock?**
    a. Metabolic acidosis
    b. Respiratory alkalosis
    c. Acute renal failure
    d. Paralytic ileus
    e. GI bleeding
    f. DIC
    g. Multiple organ failure
    h. Cardiogenic shock from the heart being overworked trying to compensate

i. Cardiac dysrhythmias

j. Death

5. What other assessment data would be helpful for the nurse to have to prepare Kevin's care plan?

a. Description of his injuries

b. MAP on admission

c. Neurological status

d. Central venous pressure

e. Presence or absence of cardiac dysrhythmias

f. Weight and height

g. Urinary output

h. Bowel sounds

i. Abdominal computed tomography or ultrasound

j. X-rays to determine presence of fractures

k. Pulse pressure

l. Arterial blood gases

m. Pulmonary artery and wedge pressures

n. Complete blood count

o. Serum electrolytes

p. Cardiac enzymes

q. Liver function tests

6. What are the priorities of care for Kevin on admission?

a. Ineffective tissue perfusion related to multiple trauma injuries

b. Risk for decreased cardiac output related to fluid loss and increased cardiac workload

c. Deficient fluid volume related to fluid loss from injuries and decreased intake

d. Ineffective protection related to decreased liver function present in shock

e. Imbalanced nutrition: less than body requirement related to NPO status and increased metabolicdemands

f. Risk for impaired skin integrity related to impaired physical mobility

g. Anxiety related to critical care environment and seriousness of Kevin's condition

h. Deficient knowledge related to Kevin's condition, treatment, and prognosis

7. Discuss the rationales for Kevin's intravenous fluid prescription.
Lactated Ringer's intravenous solution is a vascular volume expander used to rapidly increase vascular volume and tissue perfusion. In addition, the lactate ions convert to bicarbonate ions that help to reverse the metabolic acidosis present in shock. The intravenous rate will provide a liter of fluid

in 4 hours, which is higher than the normal fluid replacement or management for an 8-year-old and will provide for rapid volume expansion to increase tissue perfusion.

8.   What is the rationale for placing Kevin on mechanical ventilation? The normal respiratory rate for an 8-year-old is 16–22 breaths/minute. Kevin's rate of 45 breaths/minute will lead to exhaustion, increased insensible fluid loss, and respiratory alkalosis. By placing him on mechanical ventilation, the machine will do his work of breathing, more effectively provide oxygen to increase his oxygen saturation, and help prevent or reverse respiratory alkalosis.

9.   Discuss the purpose of the placement of Kevin's central venous access and arterial line. Kevin's central venous access provides an intravenous access that can handle the rapid infusion of intravenous fluids. In addition, it provides the means to monitor central venous pressure, an indicator of systemic fluid volume. The arterial line is placed to obtain serial arterial blood gases to monitor blood pH. This provides critical information for the development of Kevin's medical plan of care.

10.   Discuss the rationale for both continuous pulse oximetry and arterial blood gas monitoring. Although arterial blood gases provide information on oxygen saturation, the saturation is based on more central body oxygenation. In addition, the primary purpose for obtaining arterial blood gases is to monitor pH, carbon dioxide, and bicarbonate levels to determine the presence of acid–base imbalance. Pulse oximetry is noninvasive and provides information about the oxygen saturation in the periphery, a better indicator of peripheral tissue perfusion. The combined use of these two methods of monitoring is common in critical care situations.

11.   What is the health care provider's rationale for placing a nasogastric tube and an indwelling urinary catheter? The shunting of blood from the gastrointestinal tract during shock decreases peristalsis and places the client at risk for developing a paralytic ileus and the resulting risk for aspiration secondary to vomiting. The nasogastric tube is used for gastric decompression and also can be used for gastric lavage if needed in the presence of gastric bleeding. The indwelling urinary catheter is used to monitor urine output, one of the important data sources to determine the effectiveness of fluid resuscitation and renal function.

12.   Kevin's parents stay at his bedside constantly. His mother says to you, "I am so afraid my baby is not going to make it and it's all my fault. If I had just been watching the traffic closer, maybe this never would have happened." She weeps as her husband tries to console her. How can you therapeutically respond to Kevin's mother? The nurse should approach Kevin's parents with an empathetic and professional affect, allowing his mother to further express her feelings. The fact that the truck that hit her and Kevin had run a stop light as they were proceeding through the intersection indicates that the fault was with the truck driver. It is normal for parents to feel guilt when their child is injured and to chastise themselves; however, her guilt is not founded on the facts of the accident and she needs reassurance that she was not at fault. Kevin's present condition will dictate the nurse's response concerning Kevin's prognosis; however, explaining all the equipment, treatment, and rationales for his care may help to decrease her anxiety. Although Kevin's father is trying to console and support his wife, the nurse must remember that he also is experiencing anxiety, so comments should be addressed to both of them. The nurse should remind Kevin's mother that he was wearing his seat restraint that probably prevented much worse injuries.

13.   Kevin's brothers visit him regularly and even though he is not responsive, they talk to him about school and bring him cards and messages from his classmates. They bring in a CD player and play some of the current music. Discuss the potential effects of his brothers' visits. Hearing is the last sense to disappear when a client loses consciousness. The seriousness of Kevin's condition has caused him to be unresponsive; however, he may still be able to hear. The sounds of his brothers' voices and the stimulation their conversations provide for Kevin can give him a sense of familiarity and caring. The music also provides sensory stimulation to help him regain his sense of orientation when he begins to respond.

14.   Kevin's mother actively participates in his ADLs including bathing, mouth care, and range-of-motion exercises. Discuss the importance of Kevin's mother participating in Kevin's care. Her participation is important not only to Kevin but also to herself. Kevin is provided the care that he needs, and he's receiving that care by familiar and loving hands. In addition, her participation gives Kevin's mother the sense that she is doing something positive for her son, nurturing and beneficial. It also gives her time during her care to ask questions of the health care professionals. Bathing provides physical stimulation and warmth and mouth care helps to keep his oral mucous membranes moist, preventing breakdown. The range-of-motion exercises help keep his joints flexible.

15.   After Kevin has been in PICU for 1 week, his MAP is 90 mm Hg and he is being weaned from mechanical ventilation. His oxygen saturation is 100% on 30% oxygen. Discuss the significance of these findings. Tissue and organ perfusion depends on mean arterial pressure (MAP), which is the average pressure at which the blood moves through the vasculature. It is a reflection of cardiac output and peripheral resistance. An average MAP of 80–120 mm Hg is necessary to maintain cellular oxygenation and nutrition necessary to metabolize energy in amounts sufficient to sustain life.

His MAP is now within normal limits. The normal oxygen saturation is 95% to 100% so his saturation is within normal limits with supplemental oxygen. Because atmospheric oxygen concentration is 21%, his supplemental oxygen is at a low level, meaning that he is weaning from oxygen because his lungs are recovering.

16. Kevin's condition has stabilized and he is being prepared for transfer to the pediatric surgical unit. He complains of being tired and according to his parents, "He has been so cranky lately even though he's been getting better." Discuss your impression of Kevin's behavior. A client in the critical care area experiences sleep pattern disturbance as a result of the frequent assessments, noise inherent to this high stress environment and equipment, and no differentiation between day and night. Even if the client is nonresponsive, he often can still hear the voices and noises in this environment. Diagnostic testing is done 24 hours a day in critical care that also is disruptive to rest. In addition, Kevin has not been able to participate in his usual activities which can result in changes in mood. Further, Kevin may have experienced some cognitive damage as a result of the blood loss from the multiple trauma. Cognitive damage can result in personality changes in the client.

17. On the nursing unit, referrals are made to the hospital school and recreation therapy for Kevin. Discuss the rationale for these referrals. Once Kevin is transferred out of critical care, his condition is stable enough to actively engage him in activities that promote his growth and development. Obviously the facility where he is treated has a hospital school and teachers so the health care provider makes a referral to the school to help Kevin keep from getting too behind in his studies. School also is a focal part of an 8-year-old's life, providing him with opportunities for accomplishment. Recreational therapy has professionals (also may be referred to as child-life specialists) who focus on activities that promote growth and development for children of all ages who are hospitalized. These professionals have advanced educational degrees in the use of play and recreational activities as therapy. The focus of Kevin's care since his admission has been physiological, although nurses in the critical care environment provide psychosocial and spiritual care as well. Now, focusing on his growth and development becomes an important component in his recovery.

References

Broyles, B.E. (2005). *Medical-surgical nursing clinical companion.* Durham, NC: Carolina Academic Press.

Centers for Disease Control. *http://www.cdc.gov*

Chavez, J.A. and Brewer, C. (2002). Stopping the shock slide. *RN* 65(9), 30–35.

Daniels, R. (2002). *Delmar's manual of laboratory and diagnostic tests.* Clifton Park, NY: Thomson Delmar Learning.

Intravenous Therapy. *http://www.nursewise.com*

Josephson, D.L. (2004). *Intravenous infusion therapy for nurses: Principles & practice* (2nd ed.). Clifton Park, NY: Thomson Delmar Learning.

North American Nursing Diagnosis Association. (2005). *Nursing diagnoses: Definitions & classifications, 2005–2006.* Philadelphia: NANDA.

Potts, N. and Mandleco, B. (2002). *Pediatric nursing: Caring for children and their families.* Clifton Park, NY: Thomson Delmar Learning, pp. 385–387.

Pullen, R.L. (2003). Caring for a patient on pulse oximetry. *Nursing 2003* 33(9), 30.

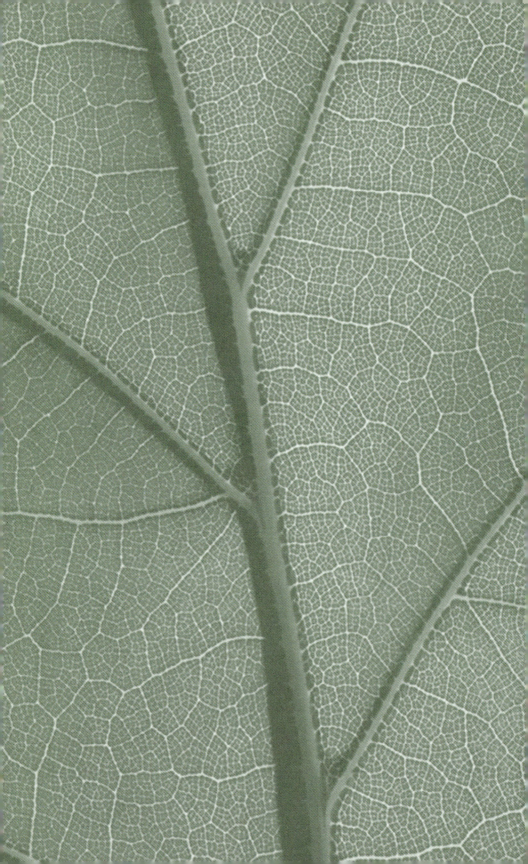

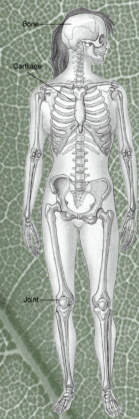

PART FOUR

Bone

Cartilage

Joint

Skeletal system
Bones, cartilage, and joints.

The Skeletal, Muscular, and Integumentary Systems

C A S E   S T U D Y   1

Kyla

GENDER

- F

AGE

8 months old

SETTING

- Hospital

ETHNICITY

- Black American

CULTURAL CONSIDERATION

PREEXISTING CONDITIONS

COEXISTING CONDITIONS

COMMUNICATION

DISABILITY

SOCIOECONOMIC

- Lower socioeconomic

SPIRITUAL

PHARMACOLOGIC

PSYCHOSOCIAL

- Single teenage mother
- Family history of abuse

LEGAL

- Mandatory reporting

ETHICAL

- Suspected abuse

ALTERNATIVE THERAPY

PRIORITIZATION

DELEGATION

THE INTEGUMENTARY SYSTEM

Level of difficulty: Easy

Overview: This case requires knowledge of burns, child abuse, as well as an understanding of the client's background, personal situation, and mother–child attachment relationship.

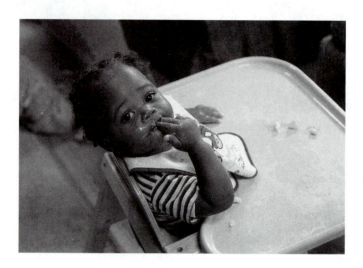

Client Profile

Kyla is an 8-month-old infant who lives with her mother, grandmother, and great grandmother in Cincinnati, Ohio. Her mother, Sierra, is a 16-year-old who stopped going to school after she became pregnant by her on-again, off-again 18-year-old boyfriend, Kyle, who visits Sierra but shows no interest in Kyla. He frequently becomes annoyed and leaves when Kyla needs to be fed or have her diapers changed. Sierra's father was very abusive to both Sierra and her mother as Sierra was growing up. He died 6 months ago as a result of a knife wound that occurred during a fight at a local tavern. He and Sierra's mother lived together with their five children and when he worked, he worked for a minimum wage that barely fed his family. Kyla's aunts and uncles (Sierra's three sisters and one brother) keep in contact with their mother and sister, but are busy with their own lives and families. Although Sierra participates in Kyla's care, her mother is the stable caregiver when she is not working. The relationship between Sierra and her mother has been strained since Sierra became pregnant and frequently the two engage in heated arguments over the increased financial stress related to Kyla's needs and Sierra's refusal to seek employment. Sierra's grandmother is in poor health and requires frequent visits to the emergency room as a result of unstable angina.

Case Study

At 2135 hours, Kyla is brought wrapped in a bath towel by her grandmother to the emergency department at the local hospital. The admitting nurse observes that Kyla is crying vigorously and is unable to be consoled. She is in no apparent respiratory distress. According to the grandmother, Kyle came over to see Sierra while Kyla's grandmother was out at the grocery. When she returned, Kyla was screaming. Sierra said that she and Kyle were talking and Kyla "got real fussy, so we decided to give her a bath to get her to quiet down, but she just kept screaming." Kyla's grandmother wrapped Kyla in a bath towel and brought her to the hospital because she thought that she was sick because "she was so red." On further assessment the nurse notes that Kyla has blisters on her feet, lower legs, and buttocks, and bruises on her upper arms. The health care provider examines Kyla and arranges for her to be transferred by AirFlight to Cincinnati Shriners' Hospital to be admitted with second-degree burns of her buttocks, genitalia, legs, and feet. Health care providers at the burn center estimate Kyla's burns as 34% of her total body surface area (TBSA) using the "Estimation of the Extent of Burns in Children" chart. Although Sierra calls every other day to ask about Kyla's condition, she doesn't visit her daughter. Kyla's grandmother stays at the hospital with Kyla.

Questions

1. Discuss your impressions about the above situation.

2. Discuss the factors in this situation that would place Kyla at risk for child abuse.

3. Using developmental theory, discuss Sierra's level of growth and development.

4. The health care providers determined that Kyla's development was appropriate for an 8-month-old infant. Discuss what you would expect when assessing Kyla's growth and development.

5. Discuss how the health care providers at the Cincinnati Shriner's Hospital arrived at 34% of Kyla's TBSA experiencing second-degree burns.

6. Describe the characteristics of second-degree burns.

7. Using the 4:2:1 rule for calculating maintenance rate of intravenous fluids for Kyla, who weighed 3.18 kg (7 lb) at birth and has experienced a weight gain within normal limits for her age, calculate her hourly IV rate.

8. Determine Kyla's priority nursing diagnoses on admission to the burn center, discussing why each is a priority.

9. Discuss your impressions about why Sierra doesn't visit Kyla at the hospital.

10. Discuss what members of the health care team should be involved in Kyla's care and recovery.

11. Discuss your feelings about child abuse and how you would feel if you were a nurse caring for Kyla in this situation.

Questions and Suggested Answers

1. Discuss your impressions about the above situation. Kyla is a normal 8-month-old infant who is the victim of child abuse. The primary concern of the health care team is to treat her injuries with a minimum of complications and report their suspicions to the legal authorities. Kyla was born into an environment where she added to the financial stress already present in this family. Her mother is an adolescent who was a victim of child abuse as well as being in a situation in which her mother also was abused. Although her father was abusive, Sierra also has had to deal with his violent death. She has dropped out of school so she doesn't have daily contact with peers, who provide the primary sense of belonging and self-esteem for an adolescent. Her teen development has been arrested by all of these factors. In addition, she may blame Kyla for her not being with her friends participating in normal adolescent activities. Sierra's grandmother also poses a stressor in this situation as Sierra must care not only for Kyla but also for her grandmother while her mother is at work. She has most likely experienced feelings of wanting to escape from this situation. Kyla still requires a great deal of care, and it is difficult for an adolescent who by normal growth and development is focused on her self and establishing her own identity to focus on the care of an infant. Kyle's presence in her life does not appear to be a healthy situation.

2. Discuss the factors in this situation that would place Kyla at risk for child abuse. Kyla was born into an environment in which abuse is the norm. Many abusers were abused themselves, as was Kyla's mother. Kyla posed additional financial stress on the family which is a characteristic of a child who is abused. Kyla's mother does not seem involved in her care as one would expect. Another characteristic of an abused child is that he or she is the product of an unwanted pregnancy. Her mother's level of growth and development also contributes to this situation because having an infant does not promote normal adolescent growth and development, which can result in resentment and anger. Kyla's father and his behavior toward Kyla also presents a potential threat.

3. Using developmental theory, discuss Sierra's level of growth and development. Sierra is an adolescent (13–20 years of age) and according to Erikson's theory, she is involved in "identity versus role confusion." During adolescence, children see themselves as distinct individuals who are unique and different from everyone else. During this time, the adolescent tends to rebel against persons she sees as authority figures. The adolescent sometimes has a confrontational relationship with the same-sex parent and is especially close to the opposite-sex parent. Risk-taking behavior (unprotected sex, smoking, drug use, speeding, etc.) is very common as the adolescent rebels against established social rules and mores. In their attempt to develop their own identity, adolescents rely primarily on peers for a sense of belonging. Consequently, behaviors are frequently the result of peer pressure. Adolescents growing up in a dysfunctional environment may "run away" as an attempt to escape this environment. According to Piaget, the adolescent is involved in formal operational thinking, allowing him or her to not only practice concrete thinking but also think about what is "possible." The adolescent is very concerned about how he or she is seen by others, especially peers. Most of the adolescent's time is spent in school and participating in school activities. Hormonal and growth changes also impact on the adolescent, with this level of growth and development being the second and final growth spurt during the lifespan. Sex hormones are secreted by the ovaries, testes, and adrenals. Menstruation begins and mood swings frequently affect adolescent personalities. Breast development occurs as well as fat deposits to fill out and contour the body, preparing it for childbearing. All of these factors contribute to this stage of growth and development being very challenging and confusing for the adolescent.

4. The health care providers determined that Kyla's development was appropriate for an 8-month-old infant. Discuss what you would expect when assessing Kyla's growth and development. Birth weight doubles in the first 6 months and triples by 1 year of age. Primary infant nutrition remains formula or breastfeeding, which should continue until 1 year of age. The addition of solid foods begins in the second 6 months of life and the infant eats six or seven times a day. An 8-month-old infant should have received the first three sets of immunizations against communicable diseases. Kyla should be sleeping 9–11 hours at night and another 4–6 hours in naps. Physically, the 8-month-old infant has lost most of the newborn reflexes (as reflexes) except Babinski (which disappears at 9 months of age), ciliary (which lasts indefinitely), and doll's eyes (which may persist into childhood). An 8-month-old can sit steadily unsupported, crawl and pull up, stand with support, and develop the pincer grasp. These infants can hold their bottles and alternate hands while feeding. Because of development in vision, they are attracted to bright colorful objects and enjoy listening to themselves make vocal sounds. They cry if in need, including the need to be held and cuddled and if anxiety is present or strangers are around.

5. Discuss how the health care providers at the Cincinnati Shriner's Hospital arrived at 34% of Kyla's TBSA experiencing second-degree burns. According to the "Estimation of the Extent of Burns in Children" chart used by many burn centers and the Shriners' facilities in particular, Kyla's burn percentage of TBSA was estimated by:

Right buttocks = 2½%
Left buttocks = 2½%
Genitalia = 1%
Right thigh = 5½%
Left thigh = 5½%
Right leg = 5%
Left leg = 5%
Right foot = 3½%
Left foot = 3½%

These represent an emersion pattern of child abuse using hot water. The percentages are adjusted according to the child's age. For an infant the rest of the TBSA estimation percentages include:

Head = 19%
Neck = 2%
Anterior trunk = 13%
Posterior trunk = 13%
Upper arm = 2½%
Lower arm = 3%
Hand = 2½%

As the child grows older and into adulthood, most of the percentages remain the same except the head percentage, which decreases with age as the thigh and leg percentages increase with age.

6. Describe the characteristics of second-degree burns. Second-degree burns are termed partial thickness burns. They are characterized by destruction of the epidermis and superficial or deep dermis with resulting loss of function (see Fig. 4-1). The loss of function depends on how much of the dermal layer is involved. Within minutes of the burn, blisters form. Fluid continues to accumulate in the blisters as the inflammatory response is triggered sending neutrophils, macrophages, basophils, and eosinophils. Phagocytosis is the key mechanisms for a successful outcome of inflammation. This process engulfs microorganisms and rids the body of debris following tissue injury. During phagocytosis, the neutrophils and macrophages adhere to the injured tissue and any microorganisms that may have entered the wound. They then ingest the cellular debris, forming a phagosome. This is followed by degradation of the debris. Superficial partial thickness burns require 7–12 days to heal as long as no infection occurs. Deep partial thickness burns require one to several months to heal and carry a higher risk of infection.

7. Using the 4:2:1 rule for calculating maintenance rate of intravenous fluids for Kyla, who weighed 3.18 kg (7 lb) at birth and has experienced a weight gain within normal limits for her age, calculate her hourly IV rate. Shriners Burn Institute (Cincinnati): 4 mL/kg per percentage burn plus 1,500 mL/m² BSA with first 8 hours—Ringer's lactate (RL) solution with 50 mEq sodium bicarbonate per liter; second 8 hours—RL solution; and third 8 hours—RL solution plus 12.5 g of 25% albumin solution per liter. Using the 4:2:1 rule for calculating maintenance rate of intravenous fluids for Kyla who weighed 3.18 kg (7 lb) at birth and has experienced a weight gain within normal limits for her age, calculate her hourly IV rate. Infants normally double their birth weight in the first 6 months and gain approximately 1 pound each month after that until 1 year of age, at which time the birth weight typically has tripled. Given Kyla's birth weight of 7 lb or 3.18 kg,

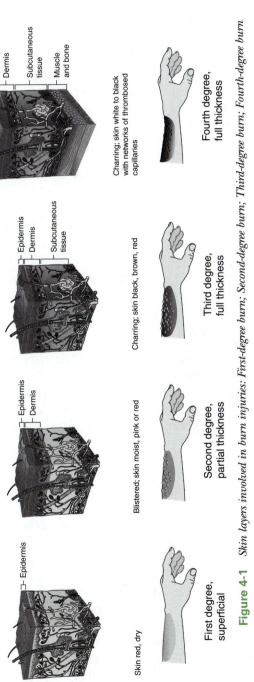

Skin red, dry

Blistered; skin moist, pink or red

Charring; skin black, brown, red

Charring: skin white to black with networks of thrombosed capillaries

Epidermis
Dermis
Subcutaneous tissue
Muscle and bone

Epidermis
Dermis
Subcutaneous tissue

Epidermis
Dermis

Epidermis

First degree, superficial

Second degree, partial thickness

Third degree, full thickness

Fourth degree, full thickness

Figure 4-1 *Skin layers involved in burn injuries: First-degree burn; Second-degree burn; Third-degree burn; Fourth-degree burn*

at 6 months her weight would be 14 lb or 6.36 kg. At 8 months her weight should be approximately 16 lb or 7.27 kg. Using the 4:2:1 rate, Kyla should receive 4 mL/kg per hour or 50.89 mL/hour.

8. Determine Kyla's priority nursing diagnoses on admission to the burn center, discussing why each is a priority.
   a. High risk of infection related to loss of skin and tissue integrity
      (1) Kyla's immune system is still immature, increasing her risk of infection secondary to the burns.
      (2) Depending on whether she experiences superficial or deep partial thickness burns, her risk of infection increases with the deeper wounds.
      (3) Being in a hospital exposes Kyla to the potential of nosocomial infection in her wounds.
   b. Acute pain related to nerve irritation at site of the burns
      (1) Second-degree burns are very painful, and considering the locations of her burns any movements of her lower extremities would create more pain.
      (2) Procedures including bathing, dressing changes, intravenous initiation, débridement (if necessary) would all be painful.
      (3) The nerve endings of newborns and infant remain very sensitive to painful stimuli because of the thinness of their skin and their acute tactile senses.
   c. Deficient fluid volume related to inflammatory process and third-spacing of fluid at burn site. Blisters filled with fluid occur almost immediately following a burn and more fluid is sent to the injury site as a result of the inflammatory process. The fluid and electrolyte balance in young children is very fragile, with imbalances occurring in these clients with much less fluid loss than it would require in an older child or adult. If the blisters lose the skin covering, fluid loss to evaporation will place them at even higher risk.
   d. Imbalanced nutrition: Less than body requirements related to nutritional demands. Nutritional requirements increase depending on the TBSA affected and the depth of the burn. A common formula used is two to three times the normal caloric intake with 23% of their nutrition in form of proteins. This usually requires some type of enteral or parenteral supplementation. If total parenteral nutrition (TPN) is needed, the presence of the central venous access device (CVAD) and the glucose content of the TPN pose further risks for infection. The use of a gastrostomy tube for enteral feedings would also increase the risk of infection.
   e. Sleep pattern disturbance related to critical care environment and frequent assessments and care. In critical care areas, assessments are

frequent 24 hours a day. Monitoring equipment involves both additional lights and sounds that can disturb sleep. If not properly managed with an opioid analgesic (morphine sulfate is the gold standard for management of moderate to severe pain in young infants, whereas fentanyl citrate may be used in children older than infants. Risk for disorganized infant behavior related to extended hospitalization and family relationships.

f. Infants are involved in Erikson's "trust versus mistrust" developmental crisis. Not having her mother with her and having her primary caregivers (nurses) change every 12 hours coupled with her normal stranger anxiety can interfere with normal development. Infants at Kyla's age are increasingly using the muscles in the legs to develop gross motor skills, which the location of her burns will at least temporarily delay. The grandmother has been the primary caregiver and is not in good health. She should be encouraged to visit and interact with Kyla whenever possible.

9. Discuss your impressions about why Sierra doesn't visit Kyla at the hospital. Sierra is probably afraid that if she visits Kyla at the hospital she may be arrested, knowing that Kyla's burns were not an accident. She may be afraid that if she visits Kyla and is questioned about Kyla's injuries, Kyle may retaliate against her. Another possible reason could be that she may be enjoying being a teenager without having an infant to care for. She may be going out with her friends or spending time with Kyle. Sierra may be having difficulty with her role as Kyla's mother and may not know how to connect with Kyla in a parent–infant relationship. We don't know whose decision it was for Sierra to keep Kyla, or whether she was coerced by other family members (her mother). Sierra may not have felt the decision was hers to make.

10. Discuss what members of the health care team should be involved in Kyla's care and recovery. *It is mandatory by law to report suspected child abuse to the appropriate child welfare agency.* Health care workers cannot return a child to a potentially abusive environment. Conclusive proof is not necessary for a person to report suspected child abuse. The laws were developed to protect children. The health care provider needs to consult with the social worker to evaluate the situation, local child welfare agent to evaluate whether it is safe to return Kyla to the home environment after recovery, local authorities to determine whether charges of child abuse should be brought against Sierra and Kyle, and recreational therapist to facilitate Kyla's growth and development and help her cope with her injuries and care.

11. Discuss your feelings about child abuse and how you would feel if you were a nurse caring for Kyla in this situation? This will involve the student addressing his or her feelings about child abuse, unwed parenthood, adolescent pregnancy, and caring for an infant with a burn injury. It also will require the student to discuss how these biases may affect care.

References

Broyles, B.E. (2005). *Medical-surgical clinical companion.* Durham, NC: Carolina Academic Press.

Burns Resuscitation and Early Management. *http://www.emedicine.com*

Cinicnnati Shriners Hospital, 3229 Burnet Avenue, Cincinnati, OH 45229-3095. (51(3) 872-6000;

FAX (51(3) 872-6999

Erikson, E.H. (1963). *Childhood and society* (2nd ed.). New York: W.W. Norton.

Gahart, B.L. and Nazareno, A.R. (2005). *2005 Intravenous medications* (21st ed.). St. Louis: Mosby.

Intravenous Therapy. *http://www.nursewise.com*

Josephson, D.L. (2004). *Intravenous infusion therapy for nurses: Principles & practice* (2nd ed.). Clifton Park, NY: Thomson Delmar Learning.

North American Nursing Diagnosis Association. (2005). *Nursing diagnoses: Definitions & classifications, 2005–2006.* Philadelphia: NANDA.

Piaget, J. (1969). *The theory of stages in cognitive development.* New York: McGraw-Hill.

Potts, N. and Mandleco, B. (2002). *Pediatric nursing: Caring for children and their families.* Clifton Park, NY: Thomson Delmar Learning.

Shriners Burn Care Hospitals: *www.schrinerhq.org*

Wong, D.L., Perry, S.E., and Hockenberry, M.J. (2002). *Maternal child nursing care* (2nd ed.). St. Louis: Mosby.

CASE STUDY 2

Triage

GENDER	**SOCIOECONOMIC**
M	
AGE	**SPIRITUAL**
5 and 8	
SETTING	**PHARMACOLOGIC**
■ Hospital/emergency department/home/clinic	
ETHNICITY	**PSYCHOSOCIAL**
■ White American	■ Anxiety
CULTURAL CONSIDERATIONS	**LEGAL**
PREEXISTING CONDITIONS	**ETHICAL**
COEXISTING CONDITIONS	**ALTERNATIVE THERAPY**
COMMUNICATION	**PRIORITIZATION**
	■ Triage situation
DISABILITY	**DELEGATION**
	■ Client teaching

MODERATE

THE SKELETAL SYSTEM

Level of difficulty: Moderate

Overview: This case requires knowledge of fractures, growth and development, as well as an understanding of the client's background, personal situation, and family–child relationship.

Client Profile

Brandon is an active 5-year-old who lives with his parents and two older siblings. He is very social and loves playing with his friends near their home. Both of his parents work, so during the school year he attends preschool and in the summer his 14-year-old sister watches him while their parents are at work. He enjoys playing with his cars and action figures and running and climbing outdoors. His father built the children a play area behind their home where Brandon does most of his outdoor activities. While their sister is in the house talking on the telephone, Brandon and his 8-year-old brother **Greg** are playing on the jungle gym and decide to climb to the top and play "King of the Mountain" even though their parents have instructed them that this game is not safe and "one of you could fall and hurt yourself." Greg climbs up first, encouraging Brandon to follow, but as Greg is reaching the top, he loses his footing and falls, knocking Brandon off the jungle gym and landing on his leg. Brandon is screaming, causing his sister to come out to see what is wrong. She finds Brandon on the ground below the jungle gym holding his left arm and Greg holding his left knee. She runs back in the house and calls her mother at work a mile from home. When their mother arrives home, Brandon is on the sofa holding his arm crying and Greg has a swollen left leg so she takes them to the emergency department of the local hospital.

Case Study

On admission, the nurse assesses Brandon and Greg. The nurse visually notes Brandon's left arm appears deformed with a bone partially protruding out of the skin. He is crying, saying his arm hurts. He is alert and oriented. His vital signs are stable although all are slightly elevated. His upper left arm reveals contusions and abrasions, and his knees also have abrasions. He also is complaining of left leg pain. Greg's knee is bruised and swollen with no breaks in the skin. His vital signs also are stable.

Questions

1. Which child requires priority care at this point?

2. Discuss the significance of Brandon's clinical manifestations.

3. Discuss the incidence and etiology of fractures in children.

4. Discuss the impact Brandon and Greg's levels of growth and development had on this situation.

5. At the scene of the accident, what are the most important interventions for Brandon?

6. Discuss fractures and their classifications and the type Brandon has based on the nurses' assessment.

7. What other assessment data are necessary for the nurse to have to prepare Brandon's care plan?

8. What are the priorities of care for Brandon on admission?

9. Discuss the potential complications if Brandon's fractures are not properly cared for at the scene of the accident or as a result of lack of care.

10. The emergency department health care provider is able to manually reduce Brandon's fracture and suture the skin wound at the site of the fracture. He applies a fiberglass brace-cast to Brandon's left arm. Discuss the rationale for applying this type of device on Brandon and the priority nursing actions following the application of Brandon's brace-cast.

11. Discuss the teaching priorities for Brandon and his mother prior to his discharge from the emergency department.

12. In 8 weeks Brandon's mother takes him to the orthopedic clinic to have his cast removed. Brandon is very quiet and cries as the nurse approaches him, clinging to his mother. Discuss your impressions of Brandon's behavior and how the nurse should respond to it.

Questions and Suggested Answers

1. Which child requires priority care at this point? Brandon appears to have a bone fracture and his skin in damaged. Greg appears to have a bruised knee rather than a fracture, as no indication is present that his knee is deformed or that he has lost skin integrity. Because of the potential complications associated with bone fractures (bleeding, compartment syndrome, nerve damage, permanent deformity, pain) and the risk of infection in the presence of loss of skin integrity, Brandon's care would take priority for the nurse. It should be noted here that Greg's care should be delegated to another nurse who is not currently in an emergency department crisis situation to address Greg's actual injuries (once diagnosed) and pain management.

2. Discuss the significance of Brandon's clinical manifestations. Brandon experienced a fall from a height sufficient to cause an open fracture of his left arm and bruises and scrapes on his left arm. His knees also have abrasions. Pain is the cardinal manifestation of a fracture. Although his exact temperature is not disclosed, the fact that it is slightly elevated may indicate infection, probably at the site of the fracture. The elevations of his other vital signs are consistent with the pain response occurring in the presence of fractures.

3. Discuss the incidence and etiology of fractures in children. Fractures are one of the most common injuries in children. Injuries from motor vehicle accidents are the most common, but in young children, fractures result from the normal activities of preschool and school-age children. Among these are fractures that result from falls. The peak incidence in childhood for fractures is at 6–9 years of age and then peaks again in adolescence. For children Brandon's age, the etiology is accidents associated with their level of growth and development combined with the porous nature of their immature bones.

4. Discuss the impact Brandon and Greg's levels of growth and development had on this situation. School-age children develop the highest level of gross motor coordination, so Greg probably is much more adept at maintaining his balance while climbing than Brandon. Brandon's gross motor skills are developing. In addition, the magical thinking associated with the preschool period can alter a preschooler's judgment related to how high an object is and his or her ability to master climbing and height. Also, it is not uncommon for a younger sibling to mimic the actions of an older sibling, especially when they are so close in age. The running, jumping, and climbing are normal activities for Brandon; however, at his age he is prone to injury as a result of these activities and his lack of coordination.

5. At the scene of the accident, what are the most important interventions for Brandon? As with any accident, the scene must be assessed to determine that it is safe for the rescuer. If the scene is safe, Brandon should be assessed for vital functions (a patent airway, breathing, and circulation) and bleeding and the actions that follow are determined by the findings of the primary survey. Brandon is alert and oriented, as evidenced by his crying. He has experienced a fall and has a deformed left arm with the bone partially protruding from the skin, which indicates an open fracture. His arm should be immobilized in the position found and transported to the nearest emergency department.

6. Discuss fractures and their classifications and the type Brandon has based on the nurse's assessment. Fractures are classified based on their characteristics and severity. The major classifications are open versus closed, simple versus compound, and complete versus incomplete. Further classifications include transverse, oblique, spiral, and greenstick (see Fig. 4-2). Open fractures involve breaks in the skin, usually with some part of the bone protruding through it. Closed fractures are beneath intact skin. Simple fractures are characterized by breaks that are uncomplicated by split off bone fragments and can usually be manually reduced. Compound fractures involve more injury to the bone and the tissues that surround the break. Complete fractures involve a total break through the entire bone, whereas with incomplete fractures, the bone remains partially intact. In transverse fractures the bone shaft is broken at a 90-degree angle. Oblique fractures involve diagonal breaks in the bone. A spiral fracture is characterized by a circular fracture line, twisting around the bone shaft. Finally, a greenstick fracture is a break through the periosteum and bone on one side with the other side of the bone intact.

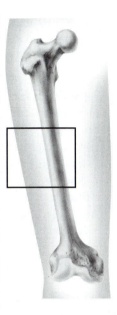

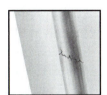

In a closed or simple fracture, the skin over the broken bone remains intact.

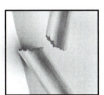

In an open or compound fracture, the broken bone protrudes through the skin.

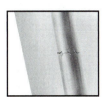

A transverse fracture occurs at a right angle to the long axis of the bone.

An oblique fracture is a slanting or diagonal break across the bone.

A spiral fracture is circular and twists around the bone shaft.

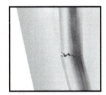

A greenstick fracture is a break through the periosteum and bone on one side while the other side only bends.

Figure 4-2 *Common childhood fractures.*

7. What other assessment data are necessary for the nurse to have to pre-pare Brandon's care plan?
   a. Radiographic studies of Brandon's left arm
   b. Magnetic resonance imaging to check the condition of the rest of his bones and tissues
   c. Complete blood count to detect bleeding or infection
   d. Computed tomography
   e. His actual vital signs
   f. Complete physical assessment

8. What are the priorities of care for Brandon on admission?
   a. Acute pain related to bone and tissue trauma
   b. Impaired skin integrity related to the trauma to the skin secondary to the fall
   c. Risk for injury, complications related to a break in the continuity of the bone, skin and nerve trauma
   d. Deficient knowledge related to Brandon's condition, treatment, and home care

9. Discuss the potential complications if Brandon's fractures are not prop-erly cared for at the scene of the accident or as a result of lack of care.
Unresolved pain is the first obvious complication that could lead to lack of use of the extremity and eventual atrophy of the muscles and contractures of the joints distal and proximal to the fracture. Compartment syndrome occurs as a result of bleeding into the muscle that surrounds the fracture.

This causes severe pain and can lead to irreversible neuromuscular damage. Attempts to reduce the fracture at the scene can lead to irreparable nerve and blood vessel damage.

10. The emergency department health care provider is able to manually reduce Brandon's fracture and suture the skin wound at the site of the fracture. He applies a fiberglass brace-cast to Brandon's left arm. Discuss the rationale for applying this type of device on Brandon and the priority nursing actions following the application of Brandon's brace-cast. A brace-cast is made of cast material; however, instead of the cast being in one piece, it is in two pieces. These types of casts are used when there is a skin injury that occurs at the site of the fracture. The fiberglass pieces are fitted and held in place with Velcro strips or a rolled bandage. This maintains the immobilization of the fracture, but also allows the health care provider to perform follow-up care on the skin wound by removing one piece of the cast to visualize the wound while keeping the other piece in place to maintain immobilization during the exam. Following the healing of the skin wound, a complete fiberglass cast is placed. The nurse must elevate Brandon's cast and extremity to decrease the edema of trauma. The cast should be handled with the palms of the hands while it is wet. Finger indentations can lead to pressure areas on the skin beneath the cast. The nurse needs to assess the skin at the proximal and distal ends of the cast to ensure that the skin is not irritated by the material. To prevent skin irritation, the cast is petaled with a soft material around the edges of the cast prior to discharge. Brandon's neurovascular status distal to the fracture and cast should be monitored to ensure no compromise or injury occurs.

11. Discuss the teaching priorities for Brandon and his mother prior to his discharge from the emergency department.
   a. Assess Brandon and his mother's current level of knowledge regarding his condition.
   b. Provide verbal and written information regarding
      (1) Accident prevention
      (2) Cast care, how to assess skin, how to promote drying of the cast, how to handle cast
      (3) Never placing anything under cast to "scratch" skin
      (4) Medication administration including proactive use of analgesics, importance of completing the prescribed medication regimen if anti-inflammatory agents or antibiotics
      (5) Signs and symptoms of adverse effects of medications
      (6) Signs and symptoms of infection, neurovascular changes
      (7) Contact phone numbers to report signs and symptoms
      (8) Importance of follow-up with health care provider and physical therapy

    c. Provide for sufficient time for Brandon and his mother to ask questions, answering them honestly.

    d. Document teaching and Brandon and his mother's response.

12. In 8 weeks Brandon's mother takes him to the orthopedic clinic to have his cast removed. Brandon is very quiet and cries as the nurse approaches him, clinging to his mother. Discuss your impressions of Brandon's behavior and how the nurse should respond to it. The stressors associated with hospitalization are evident in children undergoing what they perceive will cause them pain. Brandon remembers the pain of the fracture and associates the treatment as part of that pain experience. As long as his fracture is immobilized and healing, he should not experience discomfort. He may perceive that the removal of the cast is going to cause him pain. In addition, a preschooler's greatest stressor related to health care is the fear of mutilation. This is directly related to the child's magical thinking. He would normally ask what the cast is for following its application and the natural response to the child would involve that the cast helps his arm to heal. A preschooler would think that removal of the cast will cause him the same pain, and his arm will look as strange as it did prior to reduction and casting of the fracture. The nurse must understand growth and development and the normal perceptions of a 5-year-old. The nurse's verbalizations must be on Brandon's level of understanding, both in terms of his vocabulary and attention span (1–2 minutes/year of age) and his magical thinking. Preschoolers are very literal in their perception of words and phrases and care must be taken to avoid comments that can be misperceived by the child.

References

American Academy of Orthopaedic Surgeons. *http://www.aaos.org*

Broyles, B.E. (2005). *Medical-surgical nursing clinical companion.* Durham, NC: Carolina Academic Press.

Centers for Disease Control. *http://www.cdc.gov*

Daniels, R. (2002). *Delmar's manual of laboratory and diagnostic tests.* Clifton Park, NY: Thomson Delmar Learning.

North American Nursing Diagnosis Association. (2005). *Nursing diagnoses: Definitions & classifications, 2005–2006.* Philadelphia: NANDA.

Potts, N. and Mandleco, B. (2002). *Pediatric nursing: Caring for children and their families.* Clifton Park, NY: Thomson Delmar Learning, pp. 1138–1141.

Wong, D.L., Perry, S.E., and Hockenberry, M.J. (2002). *Maternal child nursing care* (2nd ed.). St. Louis: Mosby, pp. 1550–1555.

Felicia

GENDER

F

AGE

9

SETTING

- Hospital

ETHNICITY

- Black American

CULTURAL CONSIDERATIONS

PREEXISTING CONDITIONS

- Cerebral palsy

COEXISTING CONDITIONS

- Contractures

COMMUNICATION

- Client is nonverbal

DISABILITY

- Severe cerebral palsy

SOCIOECONOMIC

SPIRITUAL

PHARMACOLOGIC

- Oxycodone elixir (Percolone)
- Morphine sulfate (Duramorph)
- Diazepam (Valium)

PSYCHOSOCIAL

- Developmental delay

LEGAL

ETHICAL

ALTERNATIVE THERAPY

PRIORITIZATION

DELEGATION

- Client teaching

DIFFICULT

THE SKELETAL AND MUSCULAR SYSTEMS

Level of difficulty: Difficult

Overview: This case requires knowledge of cerebral palsy (CP), contractures, and surgical repair, as well as an understanding of the client's background, personal situation, and parent–child attachment relationship.

Client Profile

Felicia is an 8-year-old girl who was born with severe spastic cerebral palsy (CP) as a result of oxygen deprivation during a difficult labor and delivery. She lives at home with her parents and two older siblings. Her mother, Joyce, quit her job after Felicia was born and has provided Felicia's care at home since then. Joyce performs all of Felicia's activities of daily living (ADLs).

Case Study

Felicia is admitted to the pediatric surgical unit of the local hospital for orthopedic surgery for a femoral osteotomy and tendon lengthening for contractures. Her mother is with her and is actively involved in the admission process. Felicia is nonverbal and contracted in a fetal position.

Questions

1. What is cerebral palsy and its etiology?

2. Discuss the incidence and etiology of CP.

3. What complications are associated with Felicia's type and severity of CP?

4. What important data should the nurse collect while obtaining Felicia's admission history from Joyce?

5. What are the priorities of care for Felicia on admission?

6. Following her surgery, she is prescribed oxycodone elixir 5 mL per G-tube q6h PRN pain. Felicia cries out frequently even though she is being medicated every 6 hours with the oxycodone elixir. Her mother believes that Felicia is in pain. What is your impression of the analgesic prescription for Felicia's pain?

7. How can the nurse accurately assess Felicia's pain level?

8. The health care provider is consulted, and he prescribes morphine sulfate 1 mg continuous intravenous infusion, morphine sulfate 1 mg q1–2h intravenous bolus for breakthrough pain, and diazepam 2 mg per G-tube q6h. Felicia weighs 33 lb. Discuss the rationale for these prescriptions and determine if the doses are safe for Felicia.

9. During surgery, a spica cast was placed to facilitate immobility and healing of the surgical site. Discuss appropriate nursing interventions when caring for a child in a spica cast.

10. Discuss the teaching priorities for Felicia's mother prior to Felicia's discharge from the hospital.

Questions and Suggested Answers

1. What is cerebral palsy and its etiology? According to United Cerebral Palsy National, "'Cerebral' refers to the brain and 'palsy' to muscle weakness/poor control. Cerebral palsy itself is not progressive. . . . *It is not a disease and should not be referred to as such.*" The National Institute of Neurological Disorders and Stroke of the National Institutes of Health states, "Cerebral palsy is an umbrella-like term used to describe a group of chronic disorders impairing control of movement that appear in the first few years of life and generally do not worsen over time. The disorders are caused by faulty development of or damage to motor areas in the brain that disrupts the brain's ability to control movement and posture." It occurs in varying degree from mild to severe, reflecting the intensity of neurological deficits.

2. Discuss the incidence and etiology of CP. According to the March of Dimes, "About 2 to 3 children in 1,000 over the age of three have cerebral palsy. About 500,000 children and adults of all ages in this country have cerebral palsy." Several causative factors for CP have been identified. These include prenatal infections (rubella, cytomegalovirus, and toxoplasmosis), premature birth, insufficient oxygen to the fetus (prolapsed cord, abruptio placenta), hypoxia during labor and delivery, blood dyscrasias (Rh incompatibility, coagulation disorders), and the presence of other congenital anomalies. Head trauma is the most common cause of acquired CP.

3. What complications are associated with Felicia's type and severity of CP? Because persons with CP have damage to the motor cortex, difficulties with movement, coordination, and posture are classic complications. The extent of these complications is related to the type and severity of the CP. Felicia has severe spastic CP that results in joint and muscle deformities as a result of impaired physical mobility and spasticity. Nutritional problems occur if the child is unable to swallow. This usually requires the placement of a G-tube and enteral feedings. She is unable to perform any of her ADLs. Developmental delay is present in approximately 50% of children with CP; however, the degree of cognitive impairment varies greatly. Seizures are a frequent complication with severe CP. Sensory deficits (vision, hearing, and speech) are common, as are dental problems.

4. What important data should the nurse collect while obtaining her admission history from Joyce?
   a. How does Felicia receive nutrition? What and how often does she eat?
   b. What medications does Felicia take?
   c. Does she have seizure activity?
   d. Has she had surgery before? If so, what type and how did she respond to it?
   e. How does Felicia communicate?

    f. What is Felicia's developmental age? NOTE: Never ask if she is retarded.

    g. What is Felicia's usual routine at home?

    h. What are her urinary and bowel habits?

5. What are the priorities of care for Felicia on admission?

    a. Risk for injury related to spasms, uncontrolled movements, and possible seizures

    b. Impaired physical mobility related to spasms, joint contractures, and muscle weakness

    c. Risk for injury, seizures related to neuron irritability secondary to severe CP

    d. Delayed growth and development related to cerebral injury

    e. Impaired verbal communication related to damage to speech center and loss of coordination of facial muscles

    f. Deficient knowledge related to Felicia's surgery and postoperative course

6. Following her surgery, she is prescribed oxycodone elixir 5 mL per G-tube q6h PRN pain. Felicia cries out frequently even though she is being medicated every 6 hours with the oxycodone elixir. Her mother believes that Felicia is in pain. What is your impression of the analgesic prescription for Felicia? Felicia is probably not receiving adequate pain management considering her postoperative state. Morphine sulfate administered intravenously is the drug of choice for moderate to severe pain in children. The oxycodone elixir is generally used following 48 hours of morphine sulfate after surgery, especially following orthopedic surgery which results in high pain levels. The interval for the oxycodone elixir is too long and when it is appropriate, it should be prescribed for q4h PRN. Some health care providers mistakenly believe that children with CP do not have the same perception of pain as other children. This is a false impression, however; as a result, these children can be victims of inadequate pain control. Pain in CP children leads to the same stresses as pain in other children, including the physiological stress that interferes with healing. Another myth about pain in CP children is that if a person is unable to verbally communicate his or her pain, it is not severe. The nurse must be a client advocate and collaborate for more appropriate pain management for Felicia. Finally, concerning the myth that children receiving morphine sulfate are at high risk for respiratory depression, the nurse should share with the health care provider the rare instances of respiratory depression secondary to morphine sulfate and that as a precaution, children receiving this drug should be placed on an external cardiopulmonary monitor.

7. How can the nurse accurately assess Felicia's pain level? Felicia's mother is the best reference for the nurse in assessing Felicia's pain. With severe spastic CP, Felicia cannot verbally respond to the use of a pain assessment tool nor can she point to communicate the appropriate level. As her primary caregiver since her birth 8 years ago, Joyce knows her daughter's communication pattern better than anyone. When documenting Felicia's pain level, the nurse addresses Felicia's nonverbal pain indicators and then states, "According to Felicia's mother, Felicia is in moderate/severe pain." Following the administration of pain medication, the nurse assesses and documents Felicia's response to the intervention.

8. **The health care provider is consulted, and he prescribes morphine sulfate 1 mg continuous intravenous infusion, morphine sulfate 1 mg q1–2h intravenous bolus for breakthrough pain, and diazepam 2 mg per G-tube q6h. Felicia weighs 33 lb. Discuss the rationale for these prescriptions and determine if the doses are safe for Felicia.** As noted above, morphine sulfate is the drug of choice for pain in children. It is a highly effective Schedule II opioid analgesic. Continuous intravenous dosing provides steady pain management, avoiding the peaks and valleys of intermittent dosing. The safe dosage range of morphine is 0.1–0.2 mg/kg/dose so at 15 kg, Felicia can receive 1.5–3 mg per dose. The continuous infusion usually is one-third to one half the individual dose. The diazepam is a benzodiazepine anxiolytic that also is a potent muscle antispasmodic. Spasms will increase Felicia's pain so by treating her spasms, the analgesic will be more effective. The nurse also should find out from Felicia's mother what, if any, antispasmodic medication Felicia takes on a regular basis at home. Lorazepam is an effective alternative to diazepam. The dosing intervals are safe.

9. **During surgery, a spica cast was placed to facilitate immobility and healing of the surgical site. Discuss appropriate nursing interventions when caring for a child in a spica cast.** A spica cast is a bilateral leg cast with a bar connecting the two leg casts. This type of cast is used in children to maintain position of the surgical site and facilitates every-2-hour turning of the child. The spica cast bar should be used only to support the casts, and the child should never be lifted by the bar because it is not designed to tolerate the weight of the cast and the child's weight. Felicia's skin must be assessed every 2 hours, especially the skin at the proximal and distal ends of the cast. Neurovascular assessment also is a priority nursing intervention and should be performed with each turning. If the ends of the cast are irritating the child's skin, the casts should be petaled.

10. **Discuss the teaching priorities for Felicia's mother prior to Felicia's discharge from the hospital.** The extent of discharge teaching will depend on whether Felicia has had this type of surgery before (which is common), and if so, how much Joyce understands about Felicia's postoperative home care.

    a. Assess Joyce's level of understanding about Felicia's postoperative home care.

    b. Provide verbal and written information regarding:
       (1) Cast care including skin assessment and care
       (2) Medication administration including the importance of proactive pain management
       (3) Adverse effects of analgesic therapy (constipation) and how to prevent
       (4) Signs and symptoms of complications from surgery (infection, neurovascular compromise)
       (5) Contact phone number to report signs and symptoms
       (6) Importance of follow-up with orthopedic surgeon who performed Felicia's surgery
       (7) Referrals, as needed
    c. Joyce should be provided with sufficient time to ask questions and demonstrate understanding of how to care for Felicia and her cast.
    d. Documentation of the teaching and Joyce's response

References

Centers for Disease Control. *http://www.cdc.gov*

Gahart, B.L. and Nazareno, A.R. (2005). *2005 Intravenous medications* (21st ed.). St. Louis: Mosby.

Intravenous Therapy. *http://www.nursewise.com*

Josephson, D.L. (2004). *Intravenous infusion therapy for nurses: Principles & practice* (2nd ed.). Clifton Park, NY: Thomson Delmar Learning.

March of Dimes Birth Defects Foundation. *http://www.marchofdimes.com*

National Institute of Neurological Disorders and Stroke. *http://www.ninds.nih.gov*

North American Nursing Diagnosis Association. (2005). *Nursing diagnoses: Definitions & classifications, 2005–2006.* Philadelphia: NANDA.

Potts, N. and Mandleco, B. (2002). *Pediatric nursing: Caring for children and their families.* Clifton Park, NY: Thomson Delmar Learning, pp. 1095–1099.

Spratto, G.R. and Woods, A.S. (2005). *2005 Edition: PDR nurse's drug handbook.* Clifton Park, NY: Thomson Delmar Learning.

United Cerebral Palsy National. *http://www.upc.org*

Wong, D.L., Perry, S.E., and Hockenberry, M.J. (2002). *Maternal child nursing care* (2nd ed.). St. Louis: Mosby, pp. 1582–1587.

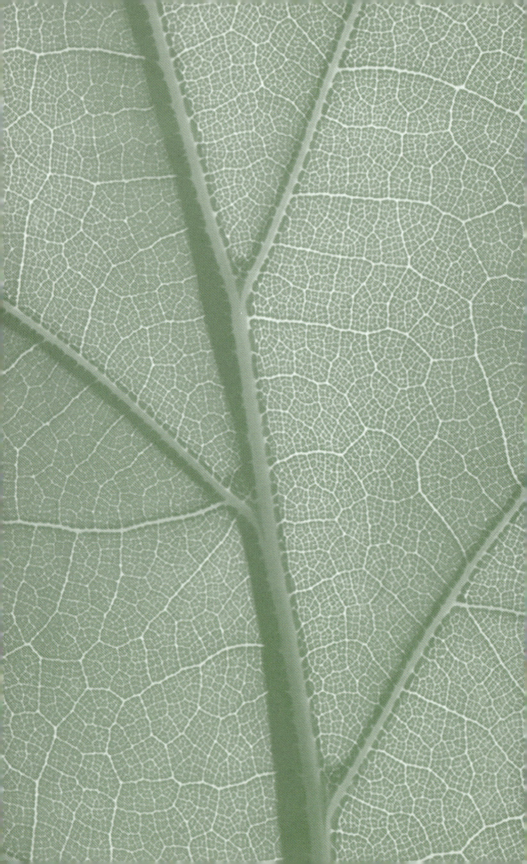

Brain

Spinal
cord

Nerves

Nervous system Brain, spinal
cord, and nerves.

The Nervous
and Endocrine
Systems

CASE STUDY 1

Isabel

GENDER	**SOCIOECONOMIC**
F	
AGE	**SPIRITUAL**
2½	
SETTING	**PHARMACOLOGIC**
■ Clinic	
ETHNICITY	**PSYCHOSOCIAL**
■ Spanish American	■ Routine exposure to cigarette smoke
CULTURAL CONSIDERATIONS	■ Parental anxiety
	LEGAL
PREEXISTING CONDITIONS	
	ETHICAL
COEXISTING CONDITIONS	■ Possible nurse bias
	ALTERNATIVE THERAPY
COMMUNICATION	
	PRIORITIZATION
DISABILITY	
	DELEGATION

THE NERVOUS SYSTEM

Level of difficulty: Easy

Overview: This case requires knowledge of otitis media, hearing impairment, the long-term effects of second-hand cigarette smoke on a child's health, growth and development, as well as an understanding of the client's background and personal situation.

Client Profile

Isabel is a 2½-year-old toddler who lives with her parents and 13-month-old sister in a rural community. Her father is a migrant worker and her mother stays at home with the children. Both parents are smokers. Both Isabel and her sister experienced recurrent episodes of otitis media during infancy although Isabel's infections have become less frequent. Isabel's speech is delayed; however, her mother believes that this is due to her lack of interactions with other children her age. Their culture and financial situation does not encourage daycare settings for children if the mother can stay at home with them. Most of Isabel's speech is not understandable although she babbles "constantly." Both children have received their scheduled immunizations at the local pediatric clinic. Isabel is brought to the clinic by her parents when she places a small toy in her ear that her parents are unable to remove.

Case Study

During the admission history, Isabel's mother tells the nurse that she has had "behavior problems" with Isabel since she was 11 months old although she stated she had not mentioned this to the staff at the clinic because she was embarrassed. On further questioning, Isabel's mother explains that Isabel "never listens to me and doesn't even look at me when I talk to her." She further states that Isabel doesn't talk so they can understand her even though they have friends whose children not only talk all the time, but she can understand what they are saying. "Isabel's problems are probably my fault because I didn't raise her right. Now I'm afraid she is retarded and I don't know how to help her." Isabel sits in her mother's lap babbling during the interview and does not make eye contact with her parents or the nurse during their conversation or when addressed. She appears disinterested in her surroundings.

Questions

1. Discuss the significance of Isabel's clinical manifestations.

2. Discuss the relationship between Isabel's history of otitis media and her present condition.

3. What is the incidence of hearing impairment in children?

4. Discuss the types of hearing impairment.

5. Discuss Isabel's mother's comment that Isabel "has always been a behavior problem" and "Isabel's problems are probably my fault because I didn't raise her right. Now I'm afraid she is retarded and I don't know how to help her."

6. What other assessment data would be helpful for the nurse to have to prepare Isabel's care plan?

7. What are the priorities of care for Isabel?

8. Discuss the effects of hearing impairment on Isabel's growth and development.

9. Discuss the standards of medical/surgical care for Isabel's hearing impairment.

10. Discuss your feelings about parents' behavior that places their children at risk.

11. How could the nurse approach Isabel's parents about their cigarette smoking and how it compromises their children?

Questions and Suggested Answers

1. Discuss the significance of Isabel's clinical manifestations. Isabel's clinical manifestations indicate that Isabel is experiencing hearing impairment, probably conductive hearing loss. Her lack of vocabulary and understandable verbalizations results from her inability to hear sounds and words to imitate. Her "behavior problems" are probably because she is unable to hear when her mother speaks to her. Frequently children with hearing impairment are mistakenly diagnosed with behavior issues because the manifestations of the two are similar including ignoring when people talk, being disinterested in what is going on around them, and inappropriate or immature language development.

2. Discuss the relationship between Isabel's history of otitis media and her present condition Recurrent otitis media is the leading cause of conductive hearing loss. With repeated infections, the middle ear structures lose their flexibility and become rigid, interfering with the conduction of sound from the environment.

3. What is the incidence of hearing impairment in children? Approximately 3 in 1,000 neonates are born with hearing impairment. Preterm infants requiring intensive or critical care have an incidence of 1% to 4% or 10–40 per 1,000 because of the immaturity of the central nervous system and sensory nerves prior to 37 weeks' gestation. In addition, nerves are the most sensitive to changes in oxygenation in the body and most preterm infants born prior to 37 weeks' gestation experience some degree of respiratory compromise and impaired gas exchange. According to Lotke, "Hearing loss occurs in 10 per 1,000 children in the United States. Of these, roughly 1 in 1,000 has profound hearing loss, and 3–5 per 1,000 have mild-to-moderate hearing loss that may affect language acquisition unless hearing and/or language are aided. Acquired hearing loss may add 10% to 20% to this figure. Internationally, sensory–neural hearing impairment occurs in 9–27 per 1,000 children."

4. Discuss the types of hearing impairment. Three types of hearing impairment have been identified: conductive, sensory–neural, and mixed (conductive and sensory–neural combined). Conductive hearing loss occurs when sound cannot be conducted through the middle ear structures. This type of hearing loss is usually mild and temporary. Sensory–neural hearing loss involves the malfunction of the cochlea in the inner ear as a result of the damage or destruction of the tiny hair cells. The term *neural* means nerve, so this type indicates damage to the auditory nerve that relays messages from the cochlea to the brain. Sensory–neural hearing loss is profound and permanent without surgical replacement of the cochlea (cochlear implant). Preterm infants of less than 37 weeks' gestation requiring intensive care following birth commonly experience this type of hearing impairment. Mixed conductive and sensory–neuron has characteristics of both types of hearing loss.

5. Discuss Isabel's mother's comment that Isabel "has always been a behavior problem" and "Isabel's problems are probably my fault because I didn't raise her right. Now I'm afraid she is retarded and don't know how to help her." Her comment about Isabel always being a behavior problem indicates that Isabel's hearing impairment has been a chronic problem probably stemming from her recurrent bouts of otitis media. Feelings of guilt are normal in parents of a child with any type of health problem. These feelings are stronger for those with children experiencing sensory deficits. Because of the perceived relationship between verbal ability and cognitive ability, concern about her child's intellectual and developmental functioning is understandable. The nurse should approach Isabel's mother in a very nonjudgmental and empathetic manner and explain that Isabel's lack of verbal skills and interest in her environment probably are related to her hearing impairment and do not necessarily indicate impairment in her cognitive ability. After collaboration with the health care provider, an intelligence test may be scheduled as a part of Isabel's assessment.

6. What other assessment data would be helpful for the nurse to have to prepare Isabel's care plan?
   a. Were Isabel's episodes of otitis media treated?
   b. How many episodes did she have?
   c. Was she ever tested for hearing impairment?
   d. Does Isabel have a referral to an audiologist?
   e. Audiography results will provide information concerning the presence and severity of Isabel's hearing impairment.
   f. What do Isabel's parents know about smoking and the increased incidence of otitis media?
   g. Do they understand the relationship between recurrent otitis media and conductive hearing loss?
   h. What is their understanding of normal growth and development?

7. **What are the priorities of care for Isabel?**
   a. Disturbed sensory perception, auditory related to hearing impairment
   b. Risk for injury related to hearing impairment and growth and development
   c. Impaired verbal communication related to hearing impairment
   d. Risk for delayed growth and development related to hearing impairment
   e. Deficient knowledge, parental related to Isabel's condition, treatment, and home care

8. **Discuss the effects of hearing impairment on Isabel's growth and development.** Verbalizations in children develop by mimicking the sounds they hear. Most children can verbally communicate their needs by age 2 years, including a vocabulary of greater than 500 words. They are talkative and verbalize constantly whether someone is listening or not. This is a time of developing autonomy, from becoming a dependent individual with limited verbal skills to a more mature and increasingly independent individual who is able to verbalize her wants and needs. This also is a time of inquisitiveness and discovery that can be hampered and even dangerous without the ability to hear. Toddlers have increased incidents of injury as a result of their inquisitiveness and limited judgment (which, of course, they don't realize). Keeping toddlers from running out in the street in front of cars is a real safety concern. For Isabel, her hearing impairment compromises her even more because she cannot hear her mother's warning or the sound of an approaching car.

9. **Discuss the standards of medical/surgical care for Isabel's hearing impairment.** Conductive hearing loss is managed with the use of a hearing aid (see Fig 5-1). This device amplifies sound. The hearing aid is adjusted to the individual child and in Isabel's case may need to be accompanied by some degree of speech therapy.

10. **Discuss your feelings about parents' behavior that places their children at risk.** Passive smoking increases the incidence of otitis media by irritating and damaging the cilia of the ear and drying the respiratory passages, increasing the risk of respiratory infections leading to otitis media. The student/reader must express his or her own feelings and biases concerning this situation and resolve that these must not interfere with nursing care.

11. **How can the nurse approach Isabel's parents about their cigarette smoking and how it compromises their children?** The nurse must approach Isabel's parents in a nonjudgmental way and provide information about the relationship between passive cigarette smoking, the incidence of otitis media, and conductive hearing loss in children. An empathetic approach

is needed because tobacco addiction is a very strong one and difficult to overcome. The nurse should encourage the parents to cease smoking together as this will increase their success and provide them with information concerning smoking cessation programs. If they don't feel they can stop smoking at this point, the nurse should encourage them not to smoke in the children's environment but rather to smoke outside of the home.

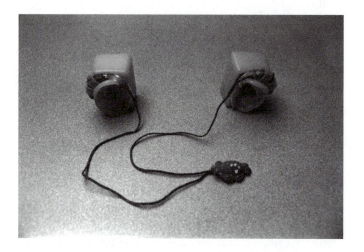

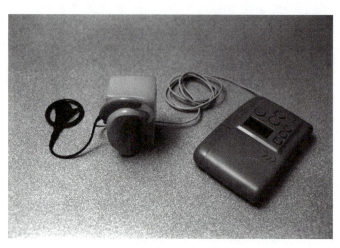

Figure 5.1 *Various types of hearing aids.*

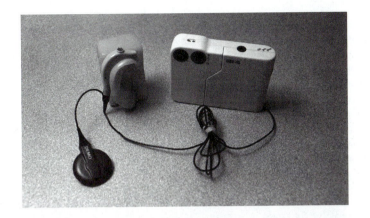

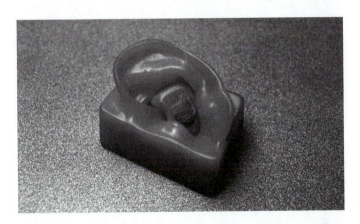

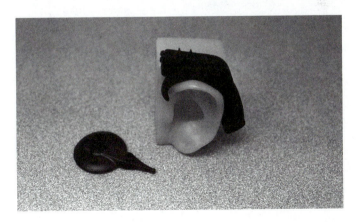

Figure 5.1 *(continued)*

References

Centers for Disease Control. *http://www.cdc.gov*

Daniels, R. (2002). *Delmar's manual of laboratory and diagnostic tests*. Clifton Park, NY: Thomson Delmar Learning.

Lotke, M. (2003). Hearing impairment. *http://www.emedicine.com*

National Library of Medicine Early identification of hearing impairment in infants and children. *http://www.nlm.nih.gov*

North American Nursing Diagnosis Association. (2005). *Nursing diagnoses: Definitions & classifications, 2005–2006*. Philadelphia: NANDA

O'Reilly, R.C. (2003). What's hearing loss. *http://www.kidshealth.org*

Potts, N. and Mandleco, B. (2002). *Pediatric nursing: Caring for children and their families*. Clifton Park, NY: Thomson Delmar Learning, pp. 1014–1023.

Wong, D.L., Perry, S.E., and Hockenberry, M.J. (2002). *Maternal child nursing care* (2nd ed.). St. Louis: Mosby, pp. 1045–1051.

CASE STUDY 2

Eugene

GENDER	**SOCIOECONOMIC**
M	■ Lower middle class
AGE	**SPIRITUAL**
4 months old	
SETTING	**PHARMACOLOGIC**
■ Hospital	■ Methadone (Dolophine)
ETHNICITY	**PSYCHOSOCIAL**
■ Black American	■ Possible delay in growth and development
CULTURAL CONSIDERATIONS	**LEGAL**
	■ Grandmother is legal guardian
PREEXISTING CONDITIONS	**ETHICAL**
■ Heroin/cocaine exposure	■ Possible nurse bias
COEXISTING CONDITIONS	**ALTERNATIVE THERAPY**
COMMUNICATION	**PRIORITIZATION**
DISABILITY	**DELEGATION**

MODERATE

THE NERVOUS SYSTEM

Level of difficulty: Moderate

Overview: This case requires knowledge of effects of fetal exposure to heroin/cocaine, growth and development, as well as an understanding of the client's background, personal situation, and mother–child attachment relationship.

Client Profile

Eugene is a 4-month-old infant living with his grandmother, who has legal guardianship of her grandson. His mother is addicted to cocaine and heroin and Eugene was exposed to these substances during gestation. He was born at 32 weeks gestation, weighing 1,364 g (3 lb). His grandmother works full-time to support herself and her grandson while Eugene attends a local daycare center. When he is at home, he spends most of his time in the playpen lying on his stomach and playing with rattles and toys suspended from strings tied to the railing of his playpen. He coos and smiles and watches his grandmother as she performs her household functions. His mother is currently a client at an inpatient detoxification center. His grandmother has taken Eugene for his scheduled appointments at the well-baby clinic since his discharge from the hospital at 6 weeks of age. He received his 2-month immunizations; however, at his 4-month follow-up, he was experiencing tachycardia, deficient weight gain, jittery episodes, irritability, and frequent "spells" of regurgitation. Because of his weight loss, he is admitted to the pediatric unit of the hospital. Each time nurses attempt to feed Eugene, he doesn't drink more than 15 mL of fluid before he falls asleep. During the feeding, the nurse notes that his suck is weak. As a result, a nasogastric tube is placed for nutritional support.

Case Study

On admission to the pediatric unit Eugene weighs 2.5 kg (5.5 lb), with oxygen saturation, 90%; temperature, 37.7° C (99.9° F); pulse, 160 beats/minute; respirations, 70 breaths/minute; and blood pressure, 70/44. Oxygen is prescribed to maintain oxygen saturation >94% and Eugene is placed on aspiration precautions, a cardiorespiratory monitor, intake and output, urine specific gravity every void, daily weights, enteral feedings of 28 calorie/ounce formula to infuse at 105 mL/hour, and methadone 0.25 mg per N/G-tube every 6 hours. His admitting diagnoses include tachycardia, failure to thrive (FTT), risk for Sudden Infant Death Syndrome (SIDS), and gastroesophageal reflux (GER).

Questions

1. Discuss the significance of Eugene's clinical manifestations.

2. Discuss the relationship between Eugene's gestational exposure to opioids and his premature birth.

3. What is the relationship between Eugene's symptoms and his premature birth?

4. What in Eugene's history places him at risk for SIDS?

5. Discuss the rationales for Eugene's admission prescriptions.

6. Discuss Eugene's methadone prescription.

7. What other medications, if any, could be used to treat Eugene's condition?

8. Considering the information you have about Eugene, discuss his level of growth and development.

9. What are the priorities of care for Eugene on admission?

10. Discuss your feelings about his mother's drug use during pregnancy.

11. Eugene has been gaining 98–105 g per day since his admission 5 days ago. His neonatal abstinence syndrome (NAS) symptoms have subsided and his grandmother is preparing to take him home. What precautions related to his risk for SIDS will Eugene's grandmother need to take when Eugene is discharged?

Questions and Suggested Answers

1. Discuss the significance of Eugene's clinical manifestations. The infant's weight indicates a deficit from the expected 1 kg (2.2 lb) per month weight gain for an infant during the first 6 months of life. Because he was 2 months premature, his growth and development will normally lag approximately 2 months less than his age until up to age 2 years. Considering his gestational exposure to heroin and cocaine, his manifestations of tachycardia, tachypnea, jitteriness, and irritability indicate neonatal abstinence syndrome (NAS). His temperature is slightly elevated, probably from the increased metabolic rate from the NAS. According to Johnson et al., (2003), "Infants exposed to certain drugs in utero may become physically dependent on them and after birth suffer withdrawal symptoms, termed the neonatal abstinence syndrome (NAS). NAS is characterized by central nervous system, gastrointestinal, and respiratory dysfunction. Affected infants commonly have irritability, high pitched cry, tremors, hypertonicity, vomiting, diarrhoea, and tachypnoea." Drugs associated with NAS include codeine, fentanyl, cocaine, heroin, methadone, meperidine, morphine sulfate, propoxyphene, caffeine, diazepam, lorazepam, diphenhydramine, marijuana, nicotine, phencyclidine, and barbiturates. His blood pressure is within normal range for his age, but it should be monitored because hypotension is a complication of premature birth.

2. Discuss the relationship between Eugene's gestational exposure to opioids and his premature birth. Premature birth and intrauterine growth retardation (IUGR) are common complications of gestational exposure to opioids. Evidence indicates that cocaine and heroin cross the placental barrier and although exactly how heroin causes IUGR is still be researched, cocaine is shown to cause infarctions in the developing organs.

3. What is the relationship between Eugene's symptoms and his premature birth? Premature infants are at risk because of physiologic immaturity of their organs and systems when born prior to the 37th week of gestation. Gastroesophageal reflux (GER) is a common complication of premature birth. The esophageal sphincter is immature and does not open and close properly. As a result, frequent regurgitation occurs that decreases nutritional intake and increases the infant's risk of aspiration and lung complications. The immaturity of the lungs due to decreased surfactant, decreased number of alveoli, smaller vessel lumens, and increased distance between the alveoli and the capillary beds creates the risk for impaired gas exchange that is evident in Eugene's tachypnea and oxygen saturation of 90%.

4. What in Eugene's history places him at risk for SIDS? According to Belik and Al-Haman (2003), "the risk for SIDS is significantly higher among infants who are exposed to opiates. Infants exposed to methadone have a 3.7-fold higher risk of SIDS in comparison to controls, whereas heroin-exposed infants have a 2.3-fold higher risk for SIDS." The nurse should collaborate with the health care provider concerning the possibility of including prescribing an apnea monitor for Eugene when he is discharged.

5. Discuss the rationales for Eugene's admission prescriptions. G-tube placement is needed to (1) decrease his risk for aspiration during oral feedings and (2) increase amount of nutrition intake without tiring the infant. The 28-calorie formula provides higher caloric intake per ounce for increased nutrition without increased volume. Continuous feedings also provide for greater nutritional intake. Aspiration precautions are appropriate because of his GER and his increased risk for SIDS. Intake and output monitoring provides objective data about Eugene's fluid balance and urine specific gravity is a measure of hydration. Daily weights monitor both nutrition and fluid balance. Cardiopulmonary monitoring is prescribed to detect abnormalities in heart and lung function on a continuous basis. This is a precaution for Eugene because of his increased risk for SIDS and his prescription for methadone, an opioid that can cause respiratory depression. Methadone is a drug used to treat the symptoms of NAS.

6. Discuss Eugene's methadone prescription. According to Johnson et al. (2003), "Morphine, diamorphine, and methadone activate opiate receptors in the locus ceruleus, one of the major clusters of noradrenergic cells in the brain. Their action decreases the activity of adenylate cyclase, resulting in a reduction in cAMP production. As a consequence, potassium efflux is increased and calcium influx into the cell is decreased, resulting in a decrease in noradrenaline (norepinephrine) release. During chronic opiate use, noradrenaline release gradually increases towards its normal level as tolerance develops. Once the opiates are withdrawn, there is loss of the inhibitory effect, and a significant increase in noradrenaline release to well above normal levels. This increase in noradrenergic activity coincides with the appearance of withdrawal symptoms in experimental models. Administration of opioids results in a reduction in neuronal activity and hence a decrease in withdrawal symptoms. Methadone and morphine have cross dependence and similar receptor effects. There are, however, potential advantages of methadone over morphine. These include better oral bioavailability, as morphine has extensive first pass metabolism, and a longer duration of action." The dosage of methadone for infants with NAS is 0.3–0.4 mg/kg every 24 hours in four divided doses. Eugene's weight is 5.5 lb, making his safe dosage range 0.75–1 mg every 24 hours or 0.1875–0.25 mg every 6 hours. NOTE: This agent is prescribed with the goal of weaning the child from it as soon as his or her condition allows.

7. What other medications, if any, could be used to treat Eugene's condition? According to Johnson, et al (2003), "Evidence suggests that opioids are the most appropriate (in the treatment of NAS), at least in infants exposed to diamorphine or methadone. In all "head to head" trials, diazepam has been shown to be ineffective. Morphine and methadone are currently the most commonly prescribed opioids to treat NAS, but randomized trials have not been undertaken to determine which is the more beneficial." Phenobarbital also is used to treat NAS at a dose of 3–6 mg/kg per day in three divided doses.

8. Considering the information you have about Eugene, discuss his level of growth and development. Infants 1–3 months of age use their hands and fingers in a grasping motion for an object. In the prone position, one could assume if Eugene grasps for objects hanging from the railing of the playpen that he can lift his head which also is characteristic of a 1- to 3-month-old infant. Smiling and cooing are consistent with the development of a 1- to 3-month-old, as is focusing and tracking noises, especially those that are consistent and familiar.

9. What are the priorities of care for Eugene on admission?
  a. Decreased cardiac output related to heart rate and oxygen saturation
  b. Impaired gas exchange related to prematurity and oxygen saturation
  c. Risk for aspiration related to history of gestational drug exposure and GER
  d. Risk for injury, SIDS related to history of gestational drug exposure
  e. Imbalanced nutrition: less than body requirements related to decreased intake
  f. Deficient knowledge related to infant's condition and health risks and needed home care

10. Discuss your feelings about his mother's drug use during pregnancy. The answer should address feelings about maternal exposure of her unborn child to illicit drugs known to cause fetal compromise. The answer also should discuss the student's/reader's understanding of the importance of identifying feelings and biases so they don't interfere with quality client care. The nurse must be able to compassionately AND objectively care for the clients as well as being a client advocate.

11. Eugene has been gaining 98–105 g per day since his admission 5 days ago. His NAS symptoms have subsided and his grandmother is preparing to take him home. What precautions related to his risk for SIDS will Eugene's grandmother need to take when Eugene is discharged? The nurse must address his grandmother's positioning of him on his stomach, as this has been associated with an increased risk of SIDS. According to the American Academy of Pediatrics, the prone position should not be used in infants until they can roll over to the position unassisted. Eugene should be placed supine or in the lateral position. In addition, with Eugene's GER, he should have his head elevated after feedings to prevent regurgitation. This can be accomplished by placing him in an infant seat in his playpen or crib for at least 30–45 minutes after each feeding. The grandmother may benefit from social worker services and child-life specialist, if available, to address financial and growth and development needs of Eugene, and a home health referral may be helpful to monitor Eugene's progress. Toys should not be suspended by strings that can break and be sources of suffocation or aspiration. Guidelines for medication administration should be provided if these prescriptions are included in Eugene's discharge prescriptions. The importance of maintaining follow-up care for Eugene must be stressed. Eugene's grandmother should have sufficient time to ask questions and obtain accurate answers prior to discharge. The teaching must be documented, including his grandmother's response to the discharge instructions.

References

American Academy of Pediatrics. *http://www.aap.org*

Belik, J. and Al-Hhamad, N. (2003). Neonatal abstinence syndrome. *http://www.emedicine.com*

Centers for Disease Control. *http://www.cdc.gov*

Johnson, K., Gerado, C., and Greenough, A. (2003). Treatment of neonatal abstinence syndrome. *http://www.fetalneonatal.highwire.org*

North American Nursing Diagnosis Association. (2005). *Nursing diagnoses: Definitions & classifications, 2005–2006.* Philadelphia: NANDA.

Wong, D.L., Perry, S.E., and Hockenberry, M.J. (2002). *Maternal child nursing care* (2nd ed.). St. Louis: Mosby, pp. 611, 650–653.

Jerod

GENDER

M

AGE

Neonate

SETTING

- Hospital

ETHNICITY

- White American

CULTURAL CONSIDERATIONS

PREEXISTING CONDITIONS

COEXISTING CONDITIONS

- Myelomeningocele

COMMUNICATION

DISABILITY

SOCIOECONOMIC

SPIRITUAL

PHARMACOLOGIC

PSYCHOSOCIAL

- Parental anxiety

LEGAL

ETHICAL

ALTERNATIVE THERAPY

PRIORITIZATION

DELEGATION

THE NERVOUS SYSTEM

Level of difficulty: Difficult

Overview: This case requires knowledge of hydrocephalus, spina bifida, growth and development, as well as an understanding of the client's background, personal situation, and parent–child attachment relationship.

DIFFICULT

Client Profile

Jerod is the name Joanna and Jim have chosen for their first child, due in 2 months. Jim has accompanied Joanna to all of her prenatal visits. During her 3-month ultrasound, they were told their baby was a boy so they have been busy preparing the nursery for his arrival. When the routine ultrasound was performed at 32 weeks' gestation, Jerod was diagnosed with hydrocephalus and a myelomeningocele. His parents were initially devastated, but remain very excited about their son's birth. Joanna is scheduled for a caesarean section at 38 weeks' gestation and the couple are very anxious about Jerod's condition and his treatment following birth.

Case Study

Jerod is delivered by caesarean section and transferred to the pediatric intensive care unit (PICU). On admission to the nursery he weighs 3.4 kg (7.5 lb) and is 8 cm (20 in.) in length. His vital signs are:

Temperature: 37° C (98.6° F)
Pulse: 144 beats/minute
Respirations: 40 breaths/minute.

He has bulging fontanels and a high-pitched cry. His head circumference is 40 cm (15.8 in.) and his chest circumference is 34 cm (13.4 in.). In the lumbar region of his spine, the nurse notes a sac-like projection. When Joanna and Jim visit the nursery, they stroke Jerod and caress his fingers and toes. Joanna begins to cry and comments to the nurse, "I so wanted to breastfeed Jerod, but now I guess I can't."

Questions

1. Discuss the reason for Jerod being delivered by caesarean section.

2. Discuss the significance of Jerod's clinical manifestations.

3. What is hydrocephalus?

4. What is a myelomeningocele and how is it related to hydrocephalus?

5. Discuss the incidence and etiology of hydrocephalus and myelomeningocele.

6. Discuss the complications associated with Jerod's myelomeningocele.

7. What are the priorities of care for Jerod on admission?

8. Discuss Jerod's parents' actions when visiting Jerod in the nursery and how the nurse should respond to Joanna's concern about breastfeeding.

9. Discuss the priority nursing interventions when caring for Jerod's myelomenigocele prior to surgery.

10. Jerod's myelomeningocele is surgically repaired and a shunt is placed for his hydrocephalus. Discuss the two types of shunts used to treat hydrocephalus and which is most common.

11. Discuss the complications that may occur in a child with a ventriculoperi-

toneal (VP) shunt and an atrioventricular (AV) shunt.

12. Discuss the teaching priorities for Jerod's parents prior to his discharge from the hospital to home.

Questions and Suggested Answers

1. Discuss the reason for Jerod being delivered by caesarean section. The decision to deliver Jerod by caesarean section was made to protect the integrity of the myelomeningocele from the stress of labor and a vaginal delivery. If he was delivered vaginally, the passage through the tight birth canal would compromise the integrity of the myelomeningocele, resulting in potential exposure of the sac contents to the vaginal canal and the air. This would increase the risk of infection and further compromise the contents of the sac, leading to additional neurological deficits for Jerod.

2. Discuss the significance of Jerod's clinical manifestations. Classic manifestations of hydrocephalus include bulging fontanels, a high-pitched cry, and an enlarged head circumference compared to the chest circumference (see Fig. 5-2). A neonate's fontanels should be flat; bulging indicates increased pressure within the brain. A high-pitched cry also is a sign of increased intracranial pressure. The head circumference of a normal neonate is within 2.5 cm (1 in.) of the chest circumference; Jerod's is 6 cm (2.4 in.) larger than his chest. This further indicates increased intracranial pressure. The sac-like projection in his lumbar region is consistent with spina bifida (see Fig. 5-3). Transillumination is a noninvasive procedure of shining a flashlight beam on the lateral aspect of the sac to determine whether the sac is filled with just fluid (meningocele) or if the sac contains solid contents (nerve roots, spinal cord, meninges, and fluid) which indicates a myelomeningocele. (Light beams can pass through fluid but not through solid tissue.) An ultrasound provides definitive differentiation, however. Jerod's vital signs are within normal limits for a neonate. Unlike in adults, vital sign indicators of increased intracranial pressure are not present in neonates until the pressure exceeds the accommodation of the flexible cranial sutures and the fontanels.

3. What is hydrocephalus? According to the National Institute of Neurological Disorders and Stroke (NINDS), "The term hydrocephalus is derived from the Greek words *hydro* meaning water and *cephalus* meaning head. As its name implies, it is a condition in which the primary characteristic is excessive accumulation of fluid in the brain. Although hydrocephalus was once known as "water on the brain," the "water" is actually cerebrospinal

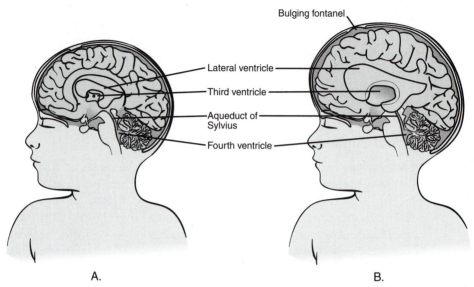

Figure 5-2 *Comparison of **A.** Normal size ventricles and
B. Enlarged ventricles associated with hydrocephalus.*

fluid (CSF)—a clear fluid surrounding the brain and spinal cord. The excessive accumulation of CSF results in an abnormal dilation of the spaces in the brain called ventricles. This dilation causes potentially harmful pressure on the tissues of the brain." Hydrocephalus is usually congenital and is associated with the following anomalies of the central nervous system:

  a. Arnold–Chiari malformation
  b. Congenital arachnoid cysts
  c. Congenital tumors
  d. Aqueduct stenosis
  e. Spina bifida (meningocele and myelomeningocele)

It also may result from conditions associated with preterm birth, neonatal meningitis, subarachnoid hemorrhage, intrauterine infection, and perinatal hemorrhage. It occurs when there is either impaired absorption of the CSF within the subarachnoid space (communicating hydrocephalus) or an obstruction of CSF flow within the ventricles, preventing CSF from entering the subarachnoid space (noncommunicating hydrocephalus).

4. **What is a myelomeningocele and how is it related to hydrocephalus?** A myelomeningocele is a congenital neural tube defect resulting from incomplete closure of the spinal column during the first 28 days of gestation. It leads to neurological deficits similar to a spinal cord injury including neurogenic bladder and bowel and weakness of the lower extremities when located in the lumbar region. Defects located higher result in more

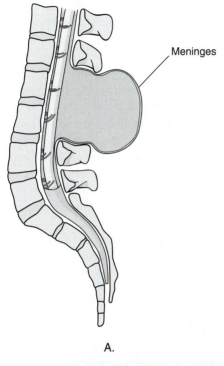

Meninges

A.

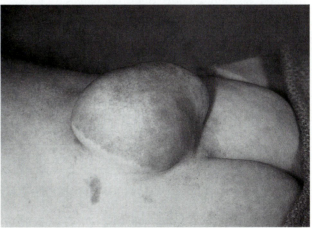

B.

Figure 5-3 *A. Illustration of meningocele;* *B. Meningocele.*

severe neurological damage including those in the thoracic level and above and may cause preterm or neonatal death. Because the central nervous system develops early, including all of its components, hydrocephalus most commonly occurs in conjunction with neural tube defects.

5. Discuss the incidence and etiology of hydrocephalus and myelomeningocele. Hydrocephalus affects approximately 1 in every 500 children, the majority occurring prenatally. The cause of hydrocephalus is not completely understood, but has been associated with genetic inheritance, complications of preterm birth, prenatal maternal infection, perinatal infection or injury, childhood tumors, or subarachnoid hemorrhage. According to the National Information Center for Children and Youth with Disabilities, "Approximately 40% of all Americans may have spina bifida occulta, but because they experience little or no symptoms, very few of them ever know that they have it." The other two types of spina bifida, meningocele and myelomeningocele, are known collectively as "spina bifida manifesta," and occur in approximately one out of every 1,000 births. Of these infants born with "spina bifida manifesta," about 4% have the meningocele form, while about 96% have myelomeningocele form. The exact cause of myelomeningocele is not known; however, evidence indicates that genetic predisposition, maternal folic acid deficiency during pregnancy, and viral infections are strongly associated with the development of spina bifida.

6. Discuss the complications associated with Jerod's myelomeningocele. Myelomeningoceles can cause life-threatening infections in the neonate if the sac loses its integrity prior to surgical closure. In addition, myelomeningocele leads to neurological deficits similar to a spinal cord injury including neurogenic bladder and bowel, weakness of the lower extremities, and paralysis when located in the lumbar region. Defects located higher result in more severe neurological damage including those in the thoracic level and above and may cause preterm or neonatal death. Because the central nervous system develops early including all of its components, hydrocephalus most commonly occurs in conjunction with neural tube defects. Latex allergies are common in these children as a result of the need for daily intermittent urinary catheterization.

7. What are the priorities of care for Jerod on admission?
    a. Ineffective cerebral tissue perfusion related to increased intracranial pressure
    b. Risk for impaired skin integrity related to fragility of myelomeningocele sac
    c. Risk for injury, neurological alterations, related to spinal cord injury
    d. Risk for infection related to potential lack of integrity of myelomeningocele sac, invasive lines, and surgical placement of shunt
    e. Risk for impaired parent/infant attachment related to Jerod's being in critical care environment
    f. Impaired urinary and bowel elimination related to interference of nerve stimulation

g. Deficient knowledge related to Jerod's condition, treatment, and home care and breastfeeding

8. How should the nurse therapeutically respond to Jerod's mother? Jerod can be breastfed. Prior to surgery, the nurse can assist Joanna in positioning Jerod on his side facing her breast, taking care not to apply any pressure to Jerod's back in the vicinity of the myelomeningocele. This position can be used postoperatively following Jerod's surgical repair and closure of the myelomeningocele. Joanna should be taught to use a breast pump to express the breast milk that can be stored in the refrigerator and administered to Jerod until the surgeon clears him for continuation of breastfeeding. The nurse should encourage Joanna about breastfeeding and her options until normal breastfeeding can continue.

9. Discuss the priority nursing interventions when caring for Jerod's myelomenigocele prior to surgery. The priority goal for the nurse is to maintain the integrity of the sac until surgery. This is accomplished by placing Jerod in a side-lying position and providing care to the sac according to the health care provider's prescription. Sac care may involve leaving the sac open to the air, applying a sterile cause dressing, a transparent dressing, or wet-to-dry dressing using sterile normal saline. Iodine substances and alcohol are very drying and should not be used on the sac. Monitoring urinary and bowel output is necessary and intermittent urinary catheterization may be prescribed to prevent bladder infections due to urinary stasis and to prevent bladder injury related to bladder distention.

10. Jerod's myelomeningocele is surgically repaired and a shunt is placed for his hydrocephalus. Discuss the two types of shunts used to treat hydrocephalus and which is most common. Ventriculoperitoneal shunts (VP shunts) are the most common type of drainage shunt used in children with hydrocephalus. This shunt functions by draining the ventricles of excess CSF and causing it to be absorbed through the peritoneal wall into systemic circulation and excreted by the kidneys. The shunt is a flexible tube beginning the ventricle and ending in the peritoneal cavity. The atrioventricular shunts (AV shunts) are much less common and are usually inserted in response to complications of the VP shunt. The AV shunt drains the ventricle(s) of the brain into the atrium of the heart to be absorbed into the blood and pumped into systemic circulation by the left cardiac ventricle. The excess fluid is then circulated systemically and excreted through the kidneys.

11. Discuss the complications that may occur in a child with a VP shunt and an AV shunt. The most common complications associated with a VP shunt are malfunction of the shunt and infection. Malfunction or obstruction of the shunt will lead to increased intracranial pressure. Infection in the shunt can lead to central nervous system infections that can lead to death.

An AV shunt can experience the same complications as a VP shunt, but with the additional life-threatening complication of cardiac dysrhythmias associated with the cardiac end of the shunt coming in contact with the myocardium and stimulating dysfunctional contractions.

12. Discuss the teaching priorities for Jerod's parents prior to his discharge from the hospital to home.

  a. Assess the understanding Joanna and Jim have about Jerod's condition and surgical treatment.

  b. Demonstrate infant care including intermittent catheterization for Jerod and allow sufficient opportunities for them to return the demonstration, evaluating their ability and providing encouragement.

  c. Demonstrate range-of-motion exercises for Jerod, as prescribed, allowing for return demonstration.

  d. Discuss signs and symptoms of increased intracranial pressure, stressing the importance of reporting these immediately to Jerod's pediatrician.

  e. Discuss skin care as prescribed.

  f. Following collaboration with health care provider, discuss referral information including Home health, National Hydrocephalus Foundation, and Social Services and contact phone numbers.

  g. Discuss signs and symptoms of infection, ensuring parents know how to take Jerod's temperature (axillary) and importance of reporting temperature elevation to the health care provider.

  h. Discuss specific discharge information prescribed by the health care provider including the importance of follow-up care.

  i. Allow sufficient time for Joanna and Jim to ask questions, ensuring these are addressed by the appropriate health care professionals.

  j. Document teaching and Joanna and Jim's responses including evaluation of their abilities to provide care demonstrated.

References

Centers for Disease Control. *http://www.cdc.gov*

Daniels, R. (2002). *Delmar's manual of laboratory and diagnostic tests.* Clifton Park, NY: Thomson Delmar Learning.

Hydrocephalus. *http://www.hydroassoc.org*

National Hydrocephalus Foundation (NHF). *http://www.hydrocephalus.org*

National Information Center for Children and Youth with Disabilities. (2004). General information about spina bifida. *http://www.nichcy.org*

National Institute of Neurological Disorders and Stroke. *http://www.ninds.nih.gov*

North American Nursing Diagnosis Association. (2005). *Nursing diagnoses: Definitions & classifications, 2005–2006.* Philadelphia: NANDA.

Potts, N. and Mandleco, B. (2002). *Pediatric nursing: Caring for children and their families.* Clifton Park, NY: Thomson Delmar Learning, pp. 1063–1068.

Wong, D.L., Perry, S.E., and Hockenberry, M.J. (2002). *Maternal child nursing care* (2nd ed.). St. Louis: Mosby, p. 1466.

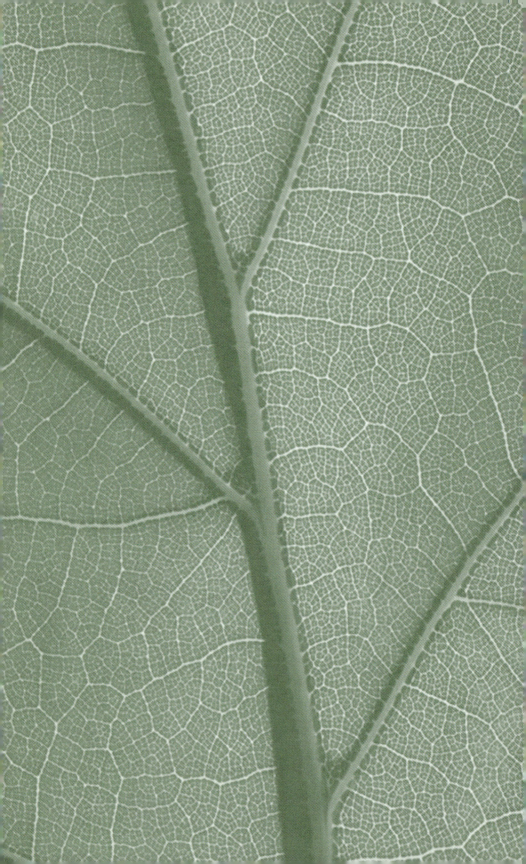

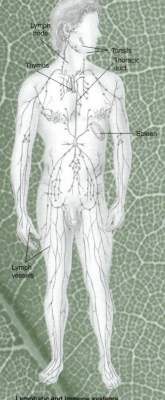

PART SIX

Lymph
node

Tonsils
Thoracic
duct

Thymus

Spleen

Lymph
vessels

Lymphatic and immune systems
Thymus, bone marrow, spleen,
tonsils, lymph nodes, lymph capillaries,
lymph vessels, lymphocytes, and lymph.

The
Lymphatic
System

Mandy

GENDER

F

AGE

4 months old

SETTING

■ Clinic

ETHNICITY

■ White American

CULTURAL CONSIDERATIONS

PREEXISTING CONDITIONS

COEXISTING CONDITIONS

COMMUNICATION

DISABILITY

SOCIOECONOMIC

■ Middle class

SPIRITUAL

PHARMACOLOGIC

■ Immunizations

■ EMLA

PSYCHOSOCIAL

■ Parental anxiety

LEGAL

■ State law requirement

ETHICAL

■ Pain management

ALTERNATIVE THERAPY

PRIORITIZATION

DELEGATION

THE LYMPHATIC SYSTEM

Level of difficulty: Easy

Overview: This case requires knowledge of immunizations, pain in infants, normal to abnormal growth and development, mother–child attachment relationship, and decision making to use EMLA prior to injection.

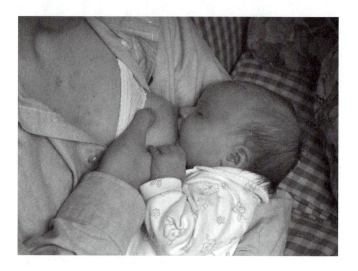

Client Profile

Mandy Dawson is a 4-month-old infant who has been in good health since birth. Her mother brings her to the Well Baby Clinic for her routine check-up. She weighed 6 lb, 2 oz at birth and is being breastfed. Her father is a manager of a retail store and her mother works outside the home. Mandy and her 3-year-old brother, Thomas, go to a local daycare center for children ages 6 weeks old to 4 years. At the conclusion of Mandy's 2-month check-up, her mother asked if anything could be done to prevent the discomfort of Mandy's immunizations. Mandy's pediatrician explains that she does not premedicate infants before immunizations although she would be willing to use ethyl chloride spray prior to the injection. Further, she states she doesn't feel it is necessary because Mandy will not remember the brief discomfort of the immunization.

Case Study

Mandy weighs 10 lb, 4 oz at this visit and appears healthy. Her mother says she is smiling and plays with her feet, often putting her foot in her mouth. She turns from her back to her abdomen and can bear weight when being held in a standing position. She reaches for objects using her palm when attempting to grasp an object.

When the nurse prepares Mandy's routine 4-month immunizations, Mandy's mother (Mrs. Dawson) states she cannot stand to see Mandy hurt and has decided against having her receive any more "shots" until something can be done so that Mandy doesn't experience pain from the shots. She further states that she is not going to bring Thomas in for any further immunizations either because he cries as soon as he enters the pediatrician's office and is inconsolable when he sees the nurse.

Questions

1. Discuss Mandy's growth and development compared to that expected of a 4-month-old infant.

2. Discuss the normal weight gain for an infant Mandy's age and compare it to Mandy's current weight.

3. What is your opinion of Mandy's mother's concern about Mandy experiencing pain during immunizations?

4. Explain whether the information given to Mandy's mother at her 2-month appointment is correct.

5. Identify the priority nursing diagnoses pertinent to this situation.

6. Discuss how the nurse could address Mandy's mother's concerns about the pain of immunizations.

7. Discuss in what way, if any, you could collaborate with the pediatrician to obtain a prescription for a local anesthetic cream or patch to apply to Mandy prior to her immunizations. Is there such a medication, is it safe for an infant Mandy's age, and how does it differ from ethyl chloride?

8. You receive a prescription of EMLA for Mandy. What is EMLA and what course of action should you take at this point?

9. Discuss what information the nurse should offer concerning the risks (including any specific risks Mandy and Thomas may have) and benefits of immunization.

10. Should you try to persuade Thomas and Mandy's mother to continue with their immunizations?

11. Discuss the procedure for administering an intramuscular injection to an infant.

12. Discuss how you could collaborate with the pediatrician to proactively prevent this situation from occurring with other mothers.

Questions and Suggested Answers

1. Discuss Mandy's growth and development compared to that expected of a 4-month-old infant. The infant's activities are appropriate for her level of growth and development. The strengthening of the abdominal muscles allows the infant to turn from a supine to a prone position. Although the infant does not have cognitive understanding, smiling begins at approximately 2 months of age in response to parents and sibling smiling at her. The fine motor skills of a 4- to 5-month-old are limited to palmar grasp.

2. Discuss the normal weight gain for an infant Mandy's age and compare it to Mandy's current weight. An infant's weight is normally double her birth weight by 6 months and triple her birth weight by 12 months. Mandy has gained 1.9 kg (4 lb, 2 oz) above her birth weight, which is a normal gain for a 4-month-old infant.

3. What is your opinion of Mandy's mother's concern about Mandy experiencing pain during immunizations? Mandy's mother's concern is valid. Intramuscular injections are painful and the site of choice for infant immunizations is the vastus lateralis muscle, which is highly innervated as well as highly vascular. The deltoid muscle is not sufficiently developed in an infant to use for intramuscular injections. Because of the close proximity of the sciatic nerve and the underdevelopment of the gluteal muscle prior to the age that the child is walking, the posterior gluteal site is unsafe for intramuscular injections and the ventral gluteal site does not contain sufficient muscle mass for immunizations.

4. Explain whether the information given to Mandy's mother at her 2-month appointment is correct. The information Mandy's mother received is only partially accurate. It is the pediatrician's prerogative to determine whether she uses a local anesthetic prior to immunizations and what agent she uses; however, the pediatrician may be uninformed about eutectic mixture of local unesthetics (EMLA) and its use in providing local anesthesia from the skin into the muscle layer when applied 1–2 hours prior to injection. Studies have shown that infants do remember painful events although not on a conscious level. The pain inflicted by immunizations also results in brief physiological effects including tachycardia, tachypnea, and hypertension.

5. Identify the priority nursing diagnoses pertinent to this situation. The priority nursing diagnoses include:

   a. Anxiety, maternal related to infant pain secondary to immunizations
   b. Acute pain related to pain of intramuscular injection secondary to immunizations
   c. Deficient knowledge related to importance of infant immunizations and availability of EMLA

6. Discuss how the nurse could address Mandy's mother's concerns about the pain of immunizations. The nurse should address the mother's concerns with empathy and understanding. She should be knowledgeable about the pain involved in intramuscular injections into the vastus lateralis muscle used for infant immunizations. She should listen to Mrs. Dawson's concerns and use therapeutic communication to encourage Mrs. Dawson to elaborate about her feelings and concerns. She also should offer suggestions for care of children at home following immunizations including applying cool compresses to the injection site and medicating the child with acetaminophen throughout the day following the injection. NOTE: According to the American Academy of Pediatrics, ibuprofen is approved as an antipyretic for children older than 6 months of age. This teaching should include safe dosages for Mandy and Thomas based on their weight. The nurse should ask Mrs. Dawson if she wants to hold Mandy for her immunizations; however, she should not be pressured into this. If she does, the nurse should explain to Mrs. Dawson how she can decrease her anxiety during the immunizations and the importance of this. The infant is perceptive of her mother's anxiety. Mrs. Dawson needs to be able to soothe and nurture her infant after any medical procedure including immunizations.

7. **Discuss in what way, if any, you could collaborate with the pediatrician to obtain a prescription for a local anesthetic cream or patch to apply to Mandy prior to her immunizations. Is there such a medication, is it safe for an infant Mandy's age, and how does it differ from ethyl chloride?** The nurse should collaborate with the pediatrician about EMLA and the safety and efficacy studies that have demonstrated its use in infants. It has been shown to be both safe and effective in preventing injection pain by anesthetizing the injection site when applied 1–2 hours prior to immunizations. Currently, pediatric nurse practitioners are working with the American Academy of Pediatrics to establish the use of EMLA as a standard of care prior to immunizations as well as other painful medical procedures. The Eutectic Mixture of Lidocaine (2.5%) and Prilocaine (2.5%) is available in both patches and cream form and when applied by the mother 1–2 hours prior to the infant's appointment supplies sufficient local anesthesia through the skin and into the muscle. It requires a prescription and many insurance companies provide payment for EMLA. Discuss the benefits of preventing painful experiences for children as well as the potential impact this could have on how children view preventative health maintenance (*http://www.aap.org*)

Ethyl chloride is used to numb the surface of the area to decrease the discomfort of the needle going through the skin. It does not have any anesthetic effect on the muscle, and many children find ethyl chloride to be painful as it is sprayed on because of how cold it feels as it is applied combined with its evaporation from the skin to the air.

8. **You receive a prescription of EMLA for Mandy. What is EMLA and what course of action should you take at this point?** Eutectic mixture of local anesthetics (EMLA) should be available in all pediatricians' offices; however, if it isn't the nurse should give the prescription to Mrs. Dawson to have filled at her pharmacy. The nurse should provide client teaching about EMLA and how and when to apply it. Choices for further action include having Mrs. Dawson apply the EMLA as soon as she receives it and have her return to the pediatrician's office after the EMLA has been applied for 2 hours. At this time Mandy can receive her immunizations. If this is not feasible, reschedule Mandy's appointment within the next 1–2 weeks and instruct Mrs. Dawson to apply the EMLA prior to that appointment time.

9. **Discuss what information the nurse should offer concerning the risks (including any specific risks Mandy and Thomas may have) and benefits of immunization.** Explain to Mrs. Dawson that the risks of immunizations are minimal including warmth, redness, and discomfort at the injection site for

6–8 hours following the immunizations. Further explain that the risks associated with contracting the diseases prevented by immunizations can be severe and even life-threatening. Review each immunization and the risks associated with each disease. Include a discussion of issues to and from other children in daycare and whether immunizations are required for children prior to attending day care.

10. Should you try to persuade Thomas and Mandy's mother to continue with their immunizations? The nurse should educate Mrs. Dawson about the importance of immunizations in preventing *Haemophilus influenzae* type B(Hib), diphtheria, pertussis, tetanus, pneumococcal conjugate (PVC), hepatitis B, influenza, and polio and stressing the risks these diseases pose for children. Mrs. Dawson appears to be genuinely interested in her children's welfare as evidenced by the fact that she has taken both her children for immunizations as scheduled. Providing her with sufficient information about both the immunizations and the ability to limit the pain associated with them should persuade Mrs. Dawson to continue with her children's immunizations.

11. Discuss the procedure for administering an intramuscular injection to an infant. An intramuscular injection for an infant requires the knowledge of the appropriate syringe size, needle size, and gauge; the appropriate site for infant injections; and the proper technique for drawing medication for a vial and administration of intramuscular injections. EMLA should be removed from the injection site using a damp cloth. Withdrawing medication from a vial includes washing hands prior to handling the equipment; inspecting the contents of the vial for clarity and the right medication, dose, and route; cleaning the cap of the vial with alcohol; injecting the amount of air equal to the amount of medication being withdrawn; and changing the needle after aspirating the medication into a 1-mL tuberculin syringe. The appropriate needle size and gauge is 5/8-inch and 25- to 27-gauge. The vastus lateralis site is the site of choice for infants and should be located using anatomical landmarks, cleansed with alcohol, and allowed to air dry. After the needle has entered the muscle, the nurse must aspirate to ensure that the needle is in the muscle and not in a vessel. After the nurse is sure of the proper placement of the needle, the medication should be slowly injected to prevent overstretching the muscle fibers which causes pain. After the injection is completed, the site should be cleansed and massaged with an alcohol swab and a small bandage applied.

12. Discuss how you could collaborate with the pediatrician to proactively prevent this situation from occurring with other mothers. The movement currently underway spear-headed by pediatric nurse practitioners is to include EMLA and the instructions on its use as a part of the going-home package new parents received prior to discharge following their child's birth. The instructions include how and when to apply the EMLA before the infant's 2-month pediatrician visit and immunizations. At this appointment the dose of EMLA needed prior to the 4-month immunizations is given to the parents with instructions. This pattern continues through the schedule of recommended childhood immunizations.

References

Managing Injection Pain. *http://www.aap.org*

Mckinney, E.S., James, S.R., Murray, S.S., and Ashwill, J.W. (2005). *Maternal-child nursing*. St. Louis: Elsevier Saunders, P. 68.

North American Nursing Diagnosis Association. (2005). *Nursing diagnoses: Definitions & classifications, 2005–2006*. Philadelphia: NANDA.

Potts, N. and Mandleco, B. (2002). *Pediatric nursing: Caring for children and their families*. Clifton Park, NY: Thomson Delmar Learning, pp. 548–550.

Reiss, B.S., Evans, M.E., and Broyles, B.E. (2002). *Pharmacological aspects of nursing care*. (6th ed.). Clifton Park, NY: Thomson Delmar Learning.

Spratto, G.R. and Woods, A.E. (2005). *2005 Edition: PDR nurse's drug handbook*. Clifton Park, NY: Thomson Delmar Learning.

Wong, D.L., Perry, S.E., and Hockenberry, M.J. (2002). *Maternal child nursing care* (2nd ed.). St. Louis: Mosby, p. 857.

C A S E   S T U D Y   2

Olasula

GENDER	**SOCIOECONOMIC**
M	
AGE	**SPIRITUAL**
4 weeks old	
SETTING	**PHARMACOLOGIC**
■ Community/hospital	
ETHNICITY	**PSYCHOSOCIAL**
■ East African	■ Parental anxiety
	■ Grief
CULTURAL CONSIDERATIONS	**LEGAL**
PREEXISTING CONDITIONS	**ETHICAL**
	■ Managing the grief process
COEXISTING CONDITIONS	**ALTERNATIVE THERAPY**
COMMUNICATION	**PRIORITIZATION**
DISABILITY	**DELEGATION**
	■ Client teaching

MODERATE

THE LYMPHATIC SYSTEM

Level of difficulty: Moderate

Overview: This case requires knowledge of HIV infection, perinatal transmission of HIV, breastfeeding, and mother–child attachment relationship.

Client Profile

Olasula is a 4-week-old infant who lives with his mother and father in the suburb of a large city. His father works and his mother stays home to care for Olasula. His father moved from Nigeria to the United States 2 years ago to attend graduate school. He regularly returned home to see his new wife who became pregnant with Olasula 6 months before moving to the United States to join her husband. The village where Olasula's parents lived has a high incidence of HIV. Olasula weighed 3.18 kg (7 lb) at birth and was 45.7 cm (18 in.) long. His mother is breastfeeding him. He required treatment for an upper respiratory infection at 2 weeks of age and is scheduled for his 4-week and follow-up visit with his pediatrician.

Case Study

Olasula's mother brings him into the pediatrician for his check-up. The infant weighs 3.4 kg (7.5 lb) and is 45.7 cm (18 in.) in length. He has a productive cough and crackles in his lower right lobe. His mother says he has not been nursing well, and she is concerned. She asks the nurse if she should change him to formula. The infant's lymph nodes in his neck and groin are enlarged, and his skin is dry. His mother further tells you that Olasula developed diarrhea last evening and has had three "dirty diapers" this morning. She describes the infant's stools as green, watery, and foul-smelling, but he has only had one wet diaper since last evening. The nurse check's the infant's oxygen saturation and finds that it is 90%.

Questions

1. Discuss your impressions about the above situation.

2. What other information would be helpful to support your impressions?

3. Discuss the incidence of HIV infections in children.

4. After the pediatrician examines the infant, he is transferred to the hospital for testing. His Western blot (for HIV antibody testing) is positive for bands and his CD4T count is 1,000 cells/mm^3. His hemoglobin is 18 g/dL and his hematocrit is 49%. His mother also is tested for HIV and her HIV antibody test results are

positive. Her CD4T count is 2,000 cells/mm^3. Discuss the significance of these diagnostic tests and results.

5. Discuss the pathophysiology of HIV.

6. What are the nursing priorities in caring for Olasula?

7. Provide opposing arguments concerning the relationship between breastfeeding and HIV infection.

8. What is the significance of Olasula's recent weight and height compared with his birth weight?

9. Could the infant's HIV have been prevented?

10. Discuss the significance of the infant's respiratory infection.

11. What treatment would you expect the health care provider to prescribe for Olasula?

12. Olasula's father expresses concern when his wife tells him that both she and Olasula are infected with HIV. He agrees to being tested and his antibody result is also positive. The nurse provides privacy and support for the parents as they experience the grief process. The nurse observes this couple being very supportive of each other. They have many questions about Olasula's condition. Discuss the nurse's role in teaching Olasula's parents about his condition.

Questions and Suggested Answers

1. **Discuss your impressions about the above situation.** When looking at Olasula's clinical manifestations and his parents' country of origin and the incidence of HIV in their home village, one should suspect that the infant was infected with HIV through prenatal or perinatal transmission. HIV rates are higher in Africa than in any other geographic area. In addition, perinatal infections occur more often in male infants than in females. His respiratory symptoms may indicate *Pneumocystis carinii* pneumonia which "accounts for 57% of AIDS-diagnoses in infants under one year (of age)" (Potts and Mandleco, 2002, 859). His history of diarrhea stools and decreased urinary output suggests that the infant probably is dehydrated.

2. **What other information would be helpful to support your impressions?**
   a. HIV antibody test. The common blood test for HIV antibodies is the Western blot assay test; however, the results require 1–2 weeks to obtain. March 26, 2004, the FDA approved the use of oral fluids samples with a rapid HIV test called OraQuick Rapid HIV-1/2 Antibody Test that is 99% accurate and supplies results in as little as 20 minutes. This would expedite the test results and allow for earlier treatment. The infant's mother also should be tested.
   b. CD4T counts for infant and mother
   c. Complete blood count
   d. Electrolyte levels
   e. Current oxygen saturation
   f. Infant's intake and output
   g. Urine specific gravity (urinalysis)
   h. Sputum culture
   i. Chest X-ray film
   j. Bronchoscopy
   k. HIV status of mother and father

3. **Discuss the incidence of HIV infections in children.** According to the Centers for Disease Control and Prevention, HIV transmission from mother

to child during pregnancy, labor, and delivery or by breastfeeding has accounted for 91% of all AIDS cases reported among U.S. children. According to the Joint United Nations Programme on HIV/AIDS, "an estimated 5 million people acquired the human immunodeficiency virus (HIV) in 2003, including 4.2 million adults and 700,000 children under 15." NOTE: The CDC statistics are based on children under 13 years old. "During 2003, AIDS caused the deaths of an estimated 3 million people, including 2.5 million adults and 500,000 children under 15. . . Today, 40 million people are estimated to be living with HIV/AIDS. Of these, 37 million are adults and 2.5 million are children under 15." Of the infants who were perinatally infected, 55% per males. More than 84% of children infected with HIV perinatally are Americans of African descent and Hispanics.

4. After the pediatrician examines the Olasula, the infant is transferred to the hospital for testing. His Western blot (for HIV antibody testing) is positive for bands and his CD4T count is 1,000 cells/mm^3. His hemoglobin is 18 g/dL and his hematocrit is 49%. His mother also is tested for HIV and her HIV antibody test results are positive. Her CD4T count is 2,000 cells/mm^3. Discuss the significance of these diagnostic tests and results. The HIV antibody test results indicate that both the infant and mother are infected with HIV. The normal CD4T count for adults is from 1,500 to 3,000/mm^3 so Olasula's mother's count shows no suppression at this time; however, Olasula's count which is normally >1,500/mm^3 indicates that he is experiencing moderate suppression. His hemoglobin and hematocrit levels are elevated. Normally these values are 9–14 g/dL and 31% to 41%, respectively. In HIV infection, these values may be decreased; however, considering the infant's diarrhea, these values when combined with the infant's history of diarrhea and decreased urinary output may indicate that he is dehydrated. The father also needs to be tested for HIV.

5. Discuss the pathophysiology of HIV. "The human immunodeficiency virus is an RNA virus in the lentivirus family and has two major strains— HIV-1 and HIV-2. Its enzyme, reverse transcriptase, is vital to its replication. HIV can be found in the blood and almost all body fluids including saliva, vaginal secretions, semen, tears, tracheal secretions, and urine" (Broyles, 2004). More than 90% of transmissions in HIV-infected infants occur prenatally or perinatally. "When the body is infected with HIV, the virus damages the cells of the immune system, specifically the CD4T lymphocytes, also called helper T cells, and causes degeneration of the central nervous system. The CD4 cells are the white blood cells that coordinate the function of the entire immune system and are necessary for humoral and cell-mediated immunity. HIV enters the cell through the cell wall and buds through the cell membrane which ultimately results in cell death. The mechanism that causes the cells to die is believed to involve the accumulation of large amounts of unintegrated viral DNA or mutated HIV envelope glyco-protein. Its initial replication occurs in the lymph nodes and plasma membrane and then gradually begins the process of cell destruction. The reduction of CD4 lymphocytes interferes with the body's ability to fight off infections caused by bacteria, viruses, and fungi. When the CD4T count falls the person becomes susceptible to opportunistic infections. These infections may be life-threatening. Furthermore, HIV causes progressive wasting disorders, including neurodegeneration, which also can result in death. Initially the body activates an anti-HIV immune response which acts to neutralize free HIV and eliminate HIV-infected cells. The anti-HIV antibody manages to inhibit the infectivity of these cells during the acute HIV infection. Anti-HIV CD8+ and cytotoxic T lymphocytes, as well as macrophages remove high numbers of circulating HIV-infected cells. This is believed to be the reason that people in the acute phases of HIV are asymptomatic. The reason for the lack of effectiveness of the natural defenses to control the long term HIV infection is not clearly understood, however it is believed to be related to the HIV's ability to use CD4 molecules as its receptor site as well as its ability to mutate and replicate. The incubation period for HIV infection to the development of AIDS is documented as being approximately 10 years. However, evidence indicates that the progression of the disease depends on how the infection was contracted. For persons who were transfused with HIV contaminated blood, the progression is much more rapid; those contaminated through a single sexual contact experience a much longer latency period for the infection to become AIDS" (Broyles, 2005).

6. **What are the nursing priorities in caring for Olasula?**
    a. Ineffective protection related to decreased CD4T count and evidence of upper respiratory infection (URI)
    b. Impaired gas exchange related to increased respiratory secretions secondary to URI
    c. Diarrhea related to the disease process
    d. Deficient fluid volume related to increased excretion of fluid secondary to diarrhea
    e. Impaired skin integrity related to excoriation from diarrhea
    f. Imbalanced nutrition related to fatigue and respiratory congestion
    g. Parental anxiety related to infant's condition
    h. Deficient knowledge related to infant's condition, treatment, prevention, and home care

7. **How would you explain to Olasula's mother the relationship between breastfeeding and HIV infection?** HIV infection can be transmitted from the mother to the breastfeeding infant at a risk as high as one in eight infants. Because HIV is transmitted through body fluids, breast milk can

transmit HIV from mother to infant. Because of advances in infant formulas, they are a very viable alternative to breastfeeding for HIV-positive mothers. "The preliminary results of the SIMBA study, reported as a late breaker at the 2nd IAS Conference on HIV Pathogenesis and Treatment in Paris, are that treating breast-fed babies with either nevirapine (NVP) or lamivudine (3TC) can greatly reduce, though not eliminate, breast milk transmission of HIV" (Meldrum, 2003).

8. What is the significance of Olasula's recent weight and height compared to his birth weight? Olasula weighed 3.18 kg (7 lb) at birth. Neonates normally lose up to 10% of their birth weight as a result of fluid loss. This weight is quickly regained and at 4 weeks the neonate has regained the weight loss as well as weight gain amounting to approximately 1.5 pounds by 4 weeks or 5–7 ounces per week. He currently weighs 3.4 kg (7.5 lb), a weight gain of 0.22 kg or less than 8 oz. Normally neonates gain approximately 2.5 cm (1 in.) in length each month for the first 6 months of life. Olasula has not grown in length since birth. His birth weight and height were within normal limits for the neonate, but he has not progressed adequately since birth. His lack of weight gain may be the result of decreased oral intake secondary to the respiratory infection as well as fluid lost through diarrhea.

9. Could the infant's HIV have been prevented? HIV transmission from mother to fetus can be prevented, but treatment has to be initiated during pregnancy. Because Olasula's mother was not aware of her HIV status, this would not have been done. Nevirapine taken during early pregnancy is the first-line antiretroviral agent of choice to prevent mother-to-fetus transmission of HIV. During pregnancy, if the mother is treated with a combination of highly active antiretroviral therapy (HAART) that suppresses the mother's viral load, transmission from mother to fetus can be prevented. The combination of nevirapine (NVP), azidothymidine (AZT), and 3TC has been shown to cross the placenta and achieve levels high enough to prevent infection in the fetus. As a result of years of research, the World Health Organization, in response to the worldwide presence of HIV, established in its 2004 report that two ART (antiretroviral therapy) regimens are safe and appropriate to use in women who are HIV positive and pregnant: d4T/3TC//NVP and ZDV/3TC/NVP. The drugs included in these regimens are lamivudine (3TC), nevirapine (NVP), stavudine (d4T), and zidovudine (ZDV), and these are considered first-line agents. With the addition of NVP to the prenatal regimen, perinatal mother-to-infant transmission has dropped significantly in industrialized countries in the past decade. The transmission rate remains higher in developing countries without knowledge or access to ARTs and HAART.

10. Discuss the significance of the infant's respiratory infection. An opportunistic microorganism that resulted from the infant's immature and compromised immune system probably caused the respiratory infection. His respiratory symptoms may indicate *Pneumocystis carinii* pneumonia (PCP), which "accounts for 57% of AIDS-diagnoses in infants under one year (of age)." (Potts and Mandleco, 2002, 859). The energy expended to fight the infection combined with the antimicrobials prescribed to treat it depleted the infant's energy stores sufficiently that he did not have the energy needed to eat. Eating is the highest energy expenditure in the neonate. In addition, the congestion in his lungs as characterized by the crackles heard by the nurse on auscultation indicate some impairment of gas exchange and this is noted in his oxygen saturation of 90%. This increases the infant's energy expenditure to breathe. Infants also lose more fluid during respirations than adults, which could increase the infant's fluid volume deficit.

11. What treatment would you expect the health care provider to prescribe for Olasula? The health care provider needs to address the infant's diarrhea and possible dehydration. Oral rehydration therapy (ORT) is the treatment of choice to treat dehydration in children; however, in infants, intravenous fluid replacement is preferred. Olasula needs to be placed on antimicrobial therapy, probably trimethoprim-sulfamethoxazole (Bactrim, Septra) which is the agent of choice for the treatment of PCP. They may augment this with a broad-spectrum antimicrobial. In treating his HIV disease, HAART is recommended by the WHO with the use of d4T or ZDV + 3TC plus EFV or NVP. The WHO further recommends that NVP be the NNRTI (non-nucleoside analog reverse transcriptase inhibitor) used in children weighing <10 kg (22 lb). Low-rate oxygen therapy will probably be prescribed during his hospitalization to increase his oxygen saturation to >94%. In addition, the health care provider may prescribe nebulizer treatments and chest physiotherapy to help increase his gas exchange and decrease the workload of breathing.

12. Olasula's father expresses concern when his wife tells him that both she and Olasula are infected with HIV. He agrees to be tested and his antibody result also is positive. The nurse provides privacy and support for the parents as they experience the grief process. The nurse observes this couple being very supportive of each other. They have many questions about Olasula's condition. Discuss the nurse's role in teaching Olasula's parents about his condition. The nurse needs to assess the parent's current level of knowledge about HIV and provide verbal and written information about Olasula's and his mother's medication regimen including the importance of strict adherence to the regimen. This information must include possible adverse effects of the medications, including the signs and symptoms of these effects, and the contact telephone numbers to report them. The nurse must provide information about infant feedings including the importance of adequate fluid intake as measured by the standard of six to eight wet diapers per day. Follow-up care for both the infant and his mother must be stressed. In addition, the nurse must provide the parents with contact numbers for any referrals prescribed. Any prescribed respiratory treatments that need to be continued at home must be explained and demonstrated (if appropriate with sufficient opportunity for the parents to return the demonstration). Also, ample time should be provided for the parents to ask questions, and the questions need to be addressed. All teaching must be documented and include the parent's response to teaching.

References

Broyles, B.E. (2005).*Medical-surgical nursing clinical companion.* Durham, NC: Carolina Academic Press.

Carter, M. (2004). *HIV & children. http://www.aidsmap.com*

Centers for Disease Control. *http://www.cdc.gov*

Daniels, R. (2002). *Delmar's manual of laboratory and diagnostic tests.* Clifton Park, NY: Thomson Delmar Learning.

Gahart, B.L. and Nazareno, A.R. (2005). *2005 Intravenous medications* (21st ed.). St. Louis: Mosby.

Joint United Nations Programme on HIV/AIDS. *http://unaids.org*

Meldrum, J. (2003). Preventing mother to child transmission of HIV. http://www.aidsmap.com

National Institute of Allergy and Infectious Diseases of National Institutes of Health. *http://www.niaid.nih.gov*

National Pediatric & Family HIV Resource Center. *http://www.pedhivaids.org*

North American Nursing Diagnosis Association. (2005). *Nursing diagnoses: Definitions & classifications, 2005–2006.* Philadelphia: NANDA.

Potts, N. and Mandleco, B. (2002). *Pediatric nursing: Caring for children and their families.* Clifton Park, NY: Thomson Delmar Learning, pp. 859–867.

Women, Children, and HIV. *http://www.womenchildrenhiv.org*

World Health Organization. *http://www.who.int*

CASE STUDY 3

Terrell

GENDER	**SOCIOECONOMIC**
M	■ Rural middle class
AGE	**SPIRITUAL**
10	■ Strength from spirituality
SETTING	**PHARMACOLOGIC**
■ Home	■ Morphine sulfate (Duramorph)
ETHNICITY	■ Hydromorphane hydrochloride (Dilaudid)
■ White American	**PSYCHOSOCIAL**
CULTURAL CONSIDERATIONS	■ Parental anxiety
	■ Grief
PREEXISTING CONDITIONS	**LEGAL**
■ Non-Hodgkin lymphoma	
COEXISTING CONDITIONS	**ETHICAL**
	■ Managing the grief process
COMMUNICATION	**ALTERNATIVE THERAPY**
DISABILITY	**PRIORITIZATION**
	DELEGATION

DIFFICULT

THE LYMPHATIC SYSTEM

Level of difficulty: Difficult

Overview: This case requires knowledge of non-Hodgkin lymphoma (NHL), as well as an understanding of death and dying (grief and grieving) and the client's background, personal situation, and family–child relationship.

Client Profile

Terrell Jones is a 10-year-old who lives with his parents and 7-year-old brother in a rural community outside a large metropolitan area. When Terrell was 6 years old, he was diagnosed with non-Hodgkin lymphoma (NHL). Following chemotherapy, Terrell achieved remission for 1 year. He then underwent chemotherapy again and eventually received a bone marrow transplant. He has been disease free for the past 3 years. Lately Terrell's parents have noted a decline in his performance at school, and he complains of nausea, indigestion, and abdominal pain. He has lost 5 pounds in the past week. His parents wonder if his immunosuppressant regimen is causing the symptoms. He begins to experience lower back and leg pain, and is too tired to play with his friends. Yesterday he developed flu-like symptoms so his mother took him to see his oncologist, who admitted him to the children's oncology unit of the research center where Terrell has received the treatments for his NHL. His parents left his younger brother with his grandmother on their way to the hospital.

Case Study

On admission, Terrell and his parents tell the nurse about Terrell's medical history and the clinical manifestations he has been experiencing. The nurse takes Terrell's vital signs and they reveal:

Temperature of 37.8° C (100° F)
Pulse: 100 beats/minute
Respirations: 30 breaths/minute
Oxygen saturation: 90%

His laboratory values include:

Hemoglobin: 9 g/dL
Hematocrit: 28%
Platelet count: 100,000/mm^3
White blood cell count: 2,500/mm^3

Bone marrow aspiration reveals the presence of lymphoma cells. A computed tomography (CT) scan shows hepatosplenomegaly. The lymph nodes in his neck, axilla, and groin are enlarged.

Questions

1. Discuss your impressions of Terrell's clinical manifestations.

2. What is the significance of Terrell's laboratory values?

3. Discuss the differences in pathophysiology between NHL and Hodgkin lymphoma.

4. What is the incidence and etiology of NHL in children?

5. Terrell is diagnosed with Stage IV NHL. Discuss the staging of NHL.

6. What are the priorities of care for Terrell on admission?

7. Terrell's pain is still not under control and he has been receiving morphine sulfate in increasing doses for 2 weeks. He is now receiving 12 mg continuous intravenous infusion and 2 mg every 8 minutes through patient-controlled analgesia (PCA) dosing. He still verbally rates his pain at 6/10. Discuss your impressions of Terrell's pain level.

8. Discuss what actions the nurse should take to assist Terrell's pain management.

9. Discuss the impact of Terrell's diagnosis on his growth and development.

10. Terrell's current relapse cannot be resolved, and the oncologist informs the family that Terrell's condition is terminal. When the nurse enters Terrell's hospital room, his mother is lying next to Terrell, weeping softly. His father and brother are sitting quietly at Terrell's bedside. As the nurse approaches the family, Terrell's father angrily says, "We did everything you told us to do, and now you say it was for nothing. How could God let this happen?" How do you explain Mr. Jones' reaction and how should the nurse respond?

11. Discuss the difference between Terrell and his brother's perception of death.

12. Terrell's parents ask what they can do to help their sons cope with the present situation.

13. Terrell receives an implanted analgesic pump and is receiving hydromorphone hydrochloride that maintains his pain level at 1–2/10 while allowing him to remain alert. He and his parents decide to take him home. Discuss Hospice and how it can benefit Terrell and his family at home.

Questions and Suggested Answers

1. Discuss your impressions of Terrell's clinical manifestations. Terrell's clinical manifestations probably indicate that Terrell has relapsed and his NHL has returned. According to the Leukemia and Lymphoma Society, nausea, indigestion, abdominal pain, weight loss, lower back pain, leg pain, fatigue, and flu-like symptoms are classical manifestations of NHL. His neck, axilla, and groin lymph nodes are enlarged. Other symptoms include vomiting, itching, headaches, bone pain, coughing, abdominal pressure, and congestion in the lymph nodes.

2. What is the significance of Terrell's laboratory values? His laboratory values may represent complications associated with immunosuppressant therapy or relapse of his NHL. The normal hemoglobin for a child his age is 11–16 g/dL. Terrell's represents anemia. The normal hematocrit for a

10-year-old is 31% to 41%. Terrell's is 28%, consistent with his hemoglobin level. His platelet count indicates thrombocytopenia as the normal range is 150,000–450,000/mm^3. His white blood cell count is only 2,500 cells/mm^3, whereas the normal is 4,100–10,800 cells/mm^3, so he is at risk for infection. His bone marrow aspiration reveals the presence of lymphoma cells and his CT scan indicates enlargement of his liver and spleen. The lymphoma cells and hepatosplenomegaly indicate NHL relapse and are not generally complications of his immunosuppressant therapy.

3. Discuss the differences in pathophysiology of NHL and Hodgkin lymphoma. One of the major differences between NHL and Hodgkin lymphoma is that Hodgkin lymphoma usually starts in the cervical lymph nodes, whereas NHL has no single point of origination. Another difference is that NHL has a very rapid onset and usually there is widespread involvement by the time it is diagnosed. Hodgkin lymphoma spreads more slowly and methodically moves from one lymph node to the next with eventual involvement in the organs if untreated. Hodgkin lymphoma also is much more responsive to chemotherapy, with longer remissions and a better prognosis because it usually is diagnosed earlier than NHL and treatment is started sooner. Both involve spread of malignant lymphocytes changing them into lymphomas. Lymphomas are acquired rather than congenital and result from damage to the DNA of lymphocytes. The damage leads to proliferation of nonfunctional lymphocytes. These crowd out the normal lymphocytes by competing for nutrients and metabolites.

4. What is the incidence and etiology of NHL in children? Approximately 9,000 children in the United States are diagnosed with cancer each year. Of these 4% are NHL and 4.4% are Hodgkin lymphoma. NHL is one and a half times more prevalent in younger children. Among adolescents, Hodgkin lymphoma is more common. The peak incidence of NHL is in children between 9 and 11 years of age. The cause of NHL is unknown; however, children with immune deficiencies (both congenital and acquired) are at higher risk of developing NHL and viral, genetic, and environmental factors may be factors in lymphoma development.

5. Terrell is diagnosed with Stage IV NHL. Discuss the staging of NHL. According to the Leukemia and Lymphoma Society, staging determines the extent of the disease. Lymphomas have four stages. Stage I means that the lymphoma is localized in either one lymph node or one organ. Stage II lymphoma indicates that two or more lymph node regions are involved. Stage III represents several lymph region involvement including the neck, chest, and abdomen. Finally, Stage IV indicates widespread involvement including the lungs, liver, intestines, and bone. Terrell's staging indicates he has the most malignant and metastatic stage of NHL. The higher the stage, the less responsive the disease is to treatment.

6. **What are the priorities of care for Terrell on admission?**
   a. Acute pain related to pressure of enlarged lymph nodes, liver, and spleen
   b. Anxiety related to Terrell's current condition
   c. Ineffective tissue perfusion related to decreased hemoglobin and hematocrit
   d. Risk for injury, infection, and bleeding related to his laboratory values
   e. Deficient knowledge related to the extent of Terrell's disease and the course of treatment needed

7. **Terrell's pain is still not under control and he has been receiving morphine sulfate in increasing dose for 2 weeks. He is now receiving 12 mg continuous intravenous infusion and 2 mg every 8 minutes through PCA dosing. He still verbally rates his pain at 6/10. Discuss your impressions of Terrell's pain level.** The intractable pain of cancer including NHL requires the use of Schedule II opioid analgesics. Morphine sulfate does not have a ceiling dose; however, the client can develop a tolerance for a given dose. Morphine sulfate is the agent of choice in children with moderate to severe pain. The general guideline for dosing is to begin with 0.1–0.2 mg/kg per dose and increase according to the child's pain level. Terrell has probably developed a tolerance for the dose of morphine sulfate.

8. **Discuss what actions the nurse should take to assist Terrell's pain management.** The nurse should assess Terrell's position to be sure it is not placing undo stress that increases pain. Once he has been positioned for comfort, the nurse must do a pain assessment. These two things should not be time consuming as Terrell is in pain. Following these actions, the nurse should collaborate with the oncologist for a further increase in the morphine dosing or a change to hydromorphone or fentanyl. Terrell's pain must be brought under control, perhaps with the addition of the anti-inflammatory agent ketorolac. Opioid analgesics work at the central nervous system level to alter perception of pain; ketorolac acts peripherally by blocking prostaglandin. By combining these agents, pain is dealt with at both levels.

9. **Discuss the impact of Terrell's diagnosis on his growth and development.** Terrell is a school-age child whose task is the development of industry versus inferiority. Industry is developed through accomplishment. Much of their sense of accomplishment occurs at school. Terrell's history of chemotherapy and a bone marrow transplant probably interfered with his attending school for periods of time. Although he obviously has excelled in his studies, another important part of his sense of accomplishment and self-esteem comes from interactions with other children his age. This is the age of "best friends" and participation in school competitive sports and other school activities.

10. Terrell's current relapse cannot be resolved, and the oncologist informs the family that Terrell's condition is terminal. When the nurse enters Terrell's hospital room, his mother is lying next to Terrell, weeping softly. His father and brother are sitting quietly at Terrell's bedside. As the nurse approaches the family, Terrell's father angrily says, "We did everything you told us to do, and now you say it was for nothing. How could God let this happen?" How do you explain Mr. Jones' reaction and how should the nurse respond? The grief response is normal in this situation and Mr. Jones's reaction is an example of grieving. The first stage is shock and denial followed by anger. When grieving, anger is a normal response in a situation where the person feels a loss of control. Often, the nurse is the object of the grief anger. This is probably because of the nurse's availability, although it may be compounded by a fear of expressing this anger to the health care provider. Bargaining is the next stage, followed by depression and then acceptance. The nurse must be an active listener with an understanding of the grief process so he or she can communicate therapeutically with this family. Terrell's family obviously needs some spiritual support at this point and this need must be addressed, perhaps by asking if they would like to speak to the hospital chaplain or contacting the family's own spiritual leader (minister, priest, rabbi) to come and see them.

11. Discuss the difference between Terrell and his brother's perception of death. At 10 years of age, Terrell has a more concrete understanding of death than his brother. At the ages of 9 and 10 years old, children understand that death is inevitable and permanent. His brother, however, still has some lingering magical thinking from his preschool age and may associate his bad behavior of thoughts as causing the situation. Further, his brother sees death as the result of the devil or a monster inside Terrell. Terrell's prognosis must be addressed with the children according to their level of growth and development and perception of the situation, reassuring them and their parents that his condition is not their fault.

12. Terrell's parents ask what they can do to help their sons cope with the present situation. The best response the nurse can give is to help the parents understand Terrell's physical and growth and development needs. The grief response should not be hurried, but rather supported. Spending time together as a family probably is very important to Terrell and should be encouraged. The nurse should collaborate with the family and the oncologist for a referral to Hospice.

13. Terrell receives an implanted analgesic pump and is receiving hydromorphone hydrochloride that maintains his pain level at 1–2/10 while allowing him to remain alert. He and his parents decide to take him home. Discuss Hospice and how it can benefit Terrell and his family at home. According to the Hospice Foundation of America, "The word "hospice" stems from the Latin word *hospitium* meaning guesthouse. It was originally used to describe a place of shelter for weary and sick travelers returning from religious pilgrimages. During the 1960s, Dr. Cicely Saunders, a British physician, began the modern hospice movement by establishing St. Christopher's Hospice near London. St. Christopher's organized a team approach to professional caregiving, and was the first program to use modern pain management techniques to compassionately care for the dying." Dr. Saunders philosophy was, "You matter until the last moment of your life, and we will do all we can, not only to help you die peacefully, but to live until you die." She introduced a focus of caring for clients so that they could die with dignity and without pain. The Foundation further notes, "Hospice is not a place but a concept of care." Hospice includes health care provider, social workers, nurses, nursing assistants, and family and spiritual care. This team works together with the family and the client to support them during the grieving and dying process. Nursing assistants can help Terrell with his activities of daily living (ADLs); the nurse assesses the client for needs such as pain medication changes, medications for constipation (a common problem for the terminally ill as a result of decreased activity, decreased intake, and the most common adverse effect of opioid analgesics required for pain management). Communication with hospice is available to the family 24 hours a day 7 days a week. To help prevent caregiver role stress, hospice can provide respite care for the family.

References

Centers for Disease Control. *http://www.cdc.gov*

Daniels, R. (2002). *Delmar's manual of laboratory and diagnostic tests.* Delmar Learning.

Gahart, B.L. and Nazareno, A.R. (2005). *2005 Intravenous medications* (21st ed.). St. Louis: Mosby.

Hospice Foundation of American. *http://www.hospicefoundation.org*

Intravenous Therapy. *http://www.nursewise.com*

Josephson, D.L. (2004). *Intravenous infusion therapy for nurses: Principles & practice* (2nd ed.). Clifton Park, NY: Thomson Delmar Learning

The Leukemia & Lymphoma Society. *http://www.leukemialymphoma.org*

North American Nursing Diagnosis Association. (2005). *Nursing diagnoses: Definitions & classifications, 2005–2006.* Philadelphia: NANDA.

Potts, N. and Mandleco, B. (2002). *Pediatric nursing: Caring for children and their families.* Clifton Park, NY: Thomson Delmar Learning, pp. 936–938.

Reiss, B.S., Evan, M.E., Broyles, B.E. (2002). *Pharmacological aspects of nursing care* (6th ed.). Clifton Park, NY: Thomson Delmar Learning, p. 246.

Wong, D.L., Perry, S.E., and Hockenberry, M.J. (2002). *Maternal child nursing care* (2nd ed.). St. Louis: Mosby, pp. 1027–1028.

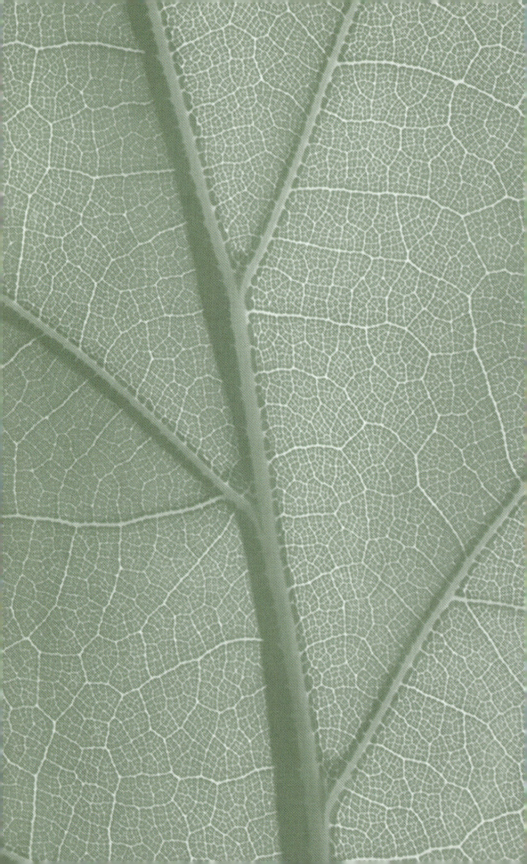

PART SEVEN

The
Reproductive
System

Mammary
gland

Ovary
Uterus
Vulva

Uterine
tube
Vagina

Reproductive systems Female;
ovaries, uterine tubes, uterus,
vagina, external genitalia, and
mammary glands.

C A S E   S T U D Y   1

Lynn

GENDER	**SOCIOECONOMIC**
F	■ Middle class
AGE	**SPIRITUAL**
15	
SETTING	**PHARMACOLOGIC**
■ Clinic	■ Doxycycline (Vibramycin)
ETHNICITY	**PSYCHOSOCIAL**
■ White American	■ Sexually active teenager
CULTURAL CONSIDERATIONS	**LEGAL**
	■ Confidentiality of minor client
PREEXISTING CONDITIONS	**ETHICAL**
COEXISTING CONDITIONS	**ALTERNATIVE THERAPY**
COMMUNICATION	**PRIORITIZATION**
DISABILITY	**DELEGATION**
	■ Client teaching

THE REPRODUCTIVE SYSTEM

Level of difficulty: Moderate

Overview: This case requires knowledge of sexually transmitted diseases (STDs), growth and development, as well as an understanding of the client's background, personal situation, and mother–child attachment relationship.

Client Profile

Lynn is a sexually active 15-year-old who lives in a suburban neighborhood with her parents and two younger sisters. She does not confide in her parents about her activities, but rather discusses them with her two best friends in high school, who also are sexually active. Last week a guest speaker at school discussed the topic of sexually transmitted diseases (STDs) which Lynn thought quite a bit about since the discussion. She has an appointment tomorrow for her annual gynecologic examination.

Case Study

In the privacy of the examination room, Lynn tells the nurse about her sexual activity and comments that her boyfriend has been experiencing a penile discharge and is concerned that "he may have infected me with some disease." When questioned by the nurse, Lynn states that she has not experienced any vaginal discharge, odor, itching, or painful intercourse. The nurse collaborates with the gynecologist who prescribes a *C. trachomatis* point-of-care test.

Questions

1. Discuss the significance of Lynn's clinical manifestations.

2. Discuss the incidence of STDs.

3. What other assessment data would be helpful for the nurse to have to prepare Lynn's care plan?

4. What are the priorities of care for Lynn during this visit?

5. Discuss the relationship between Lynn's level of growth and development and her risk for STD.

6. Lynn's *C. trachomatis* point-of-care test is positive. What does this finding mean?

7. What are the common complications associated with Lynn's condition if it is not effectively treated?

8. Lynn is prescribed doxycycline 100 mg by mouth twice a day for 7 days. Discuss your impression of this prescription.

9. Discuss the adverse effects associated with Lynn's medication prescription and the appropriate nursing actions when giving Lynn this prescription to fill.

10. Discuss Lynn's priority teaching needs prior to her discharge from the clinic.

Questions and Suggested Answers

1. Discuss the significance of Lynn's clinical manifestations. Although Lynn is asymptomatic, her boyfriend has a penile discharge. According to the Center for Disease Control and Prevention (CDC), with most STDs, the woman experiences vaginal discharge, odor, painful urination, and/or painful intercourse.

2. Discuss the incidence of chlamydia. According to the CDC, "Chlamydia is the most frequently reported bacterial sexually transmitted disease in the United States. In 2002, 834,555 chlamydial infections were reported to CDC from 50 states and the District of Columbia. Under-reporting is substantial because most people with chlamydia are not aware of their infections and do not seek testing. An estimated 2.8 million Americans are infected with chlamydia each year. Women are frequently reinfected if their sex partners are not treated.

3. What other assessment data would be helpful for the nurse to have to prepare Lynn's care plan?
  a. Vital signs
  b. How sexually active Lynn is and with how many partners
  c. Usual menstrual cycle
  d. Presence of painful urination
  e. Lynn's use of birth control
  f. Partner(s)'s use of latex condoms
  g. Results of *C. trachomatis* testing

4. What are the priorities of care for Lynn during this visit?
  a. Risk for infection, transmission related to contagious nature of STDs
  b. Risk for injury related to complications of STDs
  c. Impaired tissue integrity related to presence of pathogenic microorganisms
  d. Situational low self-esteem related to having a socially unacceptable condition
  e. Deficient knowledge related to condition, treatment, prevention of further STD

5. Discuss the relationship between Lynn's level of growth and development and her risk for STD. Adolescence is the second and final growth spurt during the life cycle. Boys gain more lean muscle mass and girls develop an increased percentage of body fat in preparation for childbirth. In addition, this is a time of hormonal changes during which girls develop breast tissue, menarche begins, and sexual maturation occurs. This is the stage of identity versus role confusion and peers are the primary source of a sense of belonging. Opposite-sex relationships become common and the pressures of peers can lead to risk-taking behaviors, among them sexual intimacy. According to the CDC, "Because the cervix . . . of teenage girls and young women is not fully matured, they are at particularly high risk for (chlamydia) infection if sexually active."

6. Lynn's *C. trachomatis* point-of-care test is positive. What does this finding mean? According to the CDC, the *C. trachomatis* point-of-care test is used to diagnose chlamydia. These tests "were developed that can be performed within 30 minutes, do not require expensive or sophisticated equipment, and are packaged as single units. The results are read qualitatively. These so-called rapid or stat tests can offer advantages in physicians' offices, small clinics and hospitals, detention centers, and other settings where results are needed immediately" so treatment can begin. Lynn's test is positive meaning she has a chlamydial infection.

7. What are the common complications associated with Lynn's condition if it is not effectively treated? According to the CDC, "If untreated, chlamydial infections can progress to serious reproductive and other health problems with both short-term and long-term consequences. Like the disease itself, the damage that chlamydia causes is often "silent." In women, untreated infection can spread into the uterus or fallopian tubes and cause pelvic inflammatory disease (PID). This happens in up to 40 percent of women with untreated chlamydia. PID can cause permanent damage to the fallopian tubes, uterus, and surrounding tissues. The damage can lead to chronic pelvic pain, infertility, and potentially fatal ectopic pregnancy. . . . Women infected with chlamydia are up to five times more likely to become infected with HIV, if exposed."

8. Lynn is prescribed doxycycline 100 mg by mouth twice a day for 7 days. Discuss your impression of this prescription. Doxycycline is among the common agents used to treat chlamydia infections. Other agents used include azithromycin 1 g by mouth in a single dose or erythromycin 500 mg by mouth q.i.d. for 7 days or erythromycin ethylsuccinate 800 mg by mouth four times a day for 10 days or ofloxacin 300 mg by mouth b.i.d. for 7 days, or levofloxacin 500 mg by mouth for 7 days. Lynn's dose, frequency, and duration of treatment is appropriate according to the CDC. The student should question whether Lynn's boyfriend also is being treated to prevent reinfection.

9. Discuss the adverse effects associated with Lynn's medication prescription and the appropriate nursing actions when giving Lynn this prescription to fill. Doxycycline is a tetracycline and the dose can be taken with meals and with a full glass of water to help prevent esophageal ulcerations. The most common adverse effect is photosensitivity so Lynn should be told to avoid such activities as sun bathing and swimming in outdoor pools until she has completed her prescription because she can easily experience a sunburn even with limited time in direct sunlight. When outdoors she should wear sunscreen. Lynn's sexual partner(s) also must be identified, tested, and treated to avoid reinfection and sexual activity should not resume until treatment is completed. However, if sexual activity does continue, latex condoms should always be used to avoid reinfection. The nurse must stress to Lynn that she take the entire prescription to avoid the development of antibiotic-resistant microorganisms.

10. Discuss Lynn's priority teaching needs prior to her discharge from the clinic.
   a. Assess Lynn's level of understanding about chlamydia
   b. Following collaboration with the health care provider, provide Lynn and her mother verbal and written instructions regarding:
      (1) CDC recommendations, "To help prevent the serious consequences of chlamydia, screening at least annually for chlamydia is recommended for all sexually active women age 25 years and younger."
      (2) Transmission of chlamydia infections (during vaginal, anal, or oral sex) and that any sexually active person is at risk for chlamydia infection as well as other STDs (assuming other STDs were ruled out) (see Fig. 7-1).

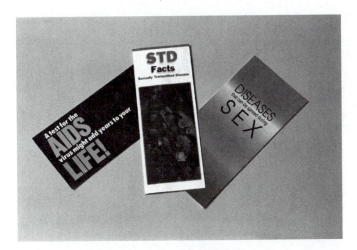

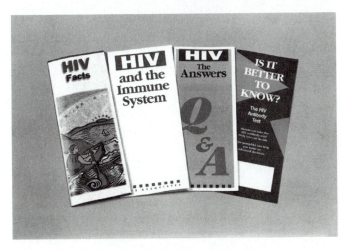

Figure 7.1   *Information on the risks of STIs, health promotion and treatment options should be provided.*

(3) Medication administration including importance of compliance with her prescription of doxycycline
(4) Signs and symptoms of adverse effects of doxycycline
(5) Signs and symptoms of worsening of condition
(6) Contact phone numbers to report signs and symptoms
(7) Importance of regular handwashing and appropriate technique
(8) Importance of follow-up with health care provider

c. Encourage Lynn to discuss her sexual activity and pregnancy prevention with her mother.
d. Provide for sufficient time for Lynn and her mother to ask questions, answering them honestly.
e. Document teaching and client and family response.

References

Centers for Disease Control. *http://www.cdc.gov*
Daniels, R. (2002). *Delmar's manual of laboratory and diagnostic tests*. Delmar Learning.
North American Nursing Diagnosis Association. (2005). *Nursing diagnoses: Definitions & classifications, 2005–2006*. Philadelphia: NANDA.
Stratto, G.R. and Woods, A.L. (2005). *2005 Edition: PDR Nurse's drug handbook*. Clifton Park, NY: Thomson Delmar Learning, pp. 584–586.

Index

Page numbers in *italic* indicate figures.